THE
PVC
DIET

THE
PVC
DIET

A simple nutritional solution

Lawrence R. Kosinski, MD, MBA

with co-author Joan Kanute, MS, RD

Contributions by:
Danielle Sell

Edited by:
Joel Brill, MD

authorHOUSE®

AuthorHouse™
1663 Liberty Drive
Bloomington, IN 47403
www.authorhouse.com
Phone: 1-800-839-8640

Published by AuthorHouse   03/12/2013

ISBN: 978-1-4817-1942-1 (sc)
ISBN: 978-1-4817-1941-4 (e)

Library of Congress Control Number: 2013903194

Contents

For Amelia

Acknowledgements

Although this book represents the longstanding compilation of many years of my medical practice, it couldn't have been put into this form without the assistance of multiple individuals.

Special thanks to the following friends and colleagues for their honest and helpful feedback: Annika Drosos; Robert H. Eltzholtz; Kathleen K. Foley, BSN, MBA; Cory Ann Martin; Deborah S. Pitlik, EdD; and Dale Reiff.

Our gracious thanks to Stacy Hadley who designed the cover art.

My long term colleague and friend, Joel Brill, MD, was instrumental in keeping me on message and in appropriate form. He is responsible for continually editing this book. I greatly appreciate his help and mentorship.

Introduction

I'm a physician who has been in private practice for over 25 years. You can imagine how many patients I have seen in over a quarter of a century. My medical specialty is Gastroenterology (GI), which means patients come to see me when they have problems in their gut or digestive tract. These are typically conditions like acid reflux (gastroesophageal reflux disease), stomach and duodenal ulcers, Celiac disease, diverticulosis, irritable bowel syndrome (IBS), colon polyps, Crohn's disease, ulcerative colitis, hepatitis, pancreatitis, cancers and other conditions. In my specialty, I see the entire spectrum of digestive diseases.

Since so many GI conditions are affected by diet, much of my office time is spent counseling patients on appropriate eating habits. In the course of a typical day, I discuss diet and nutrition with at least half of my patients. The great majority of these discussions concern their excess weight. For most physicians this is a common topic, as two-thirds of the American population is overweight, meaning their Body Mass Index (BMI) is over 25. One-third of the population is obese with a BMI over 30. Obesity is a major health issue. Counseling patients on weight reduction is extremely important since weight is intricately related to good health.

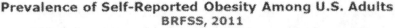

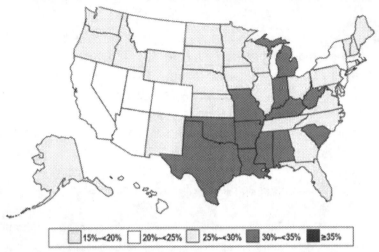

Figure: "Adult Obesity Facts," Centers for Disease Control and Prevention, updated August 2012, http://www.cdc.gov/obesity/data/adult.html

Because of aging Baby Boomers, we're also facing a "Silver Tsunami:"

- The number of people over 65 will double in the next 20 years.
- There are 10,000 new Medicare beneficiaries every day.
- Currently, 40 million seniors make up 30 percent of the U.S. population. By 2030, this will grow to 72 million seniors.
- Obesity in the senior population is way up: 38 percent of seniors were obese in 2009-2010, compared with 22 percent in 1988-1994.

In the aggregate, over 60 percent of American adults weigh more than is healthy. It costs our nation roughly $147 billion each year in medical expenses for the direct treatment of obesity and for the treatment of obesity-related diseases.

The reason for this expense is that people who are overweight are at-risk for serious diseases including heart disease, high blood pressure and diabetes which commonly occur together. The combination of these three conditions represents the Metabolic Syndrome which affects 25 percent of the population. These three disorders are clearly related. There is a direct reason for this.

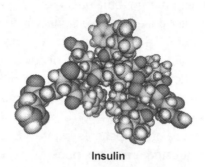

Insulin

Excess fat has an effect on the hormone insulin, which is supposed to control your blood sugar. When we ingest sugar, our pancreas secretes insulin. Insulin's job is to move the sugar and the fat out of the bloodstream and into our cells where it can be used for energy. Unfortunately, excess total body fat causes insulin to lose some of its effectiveness. If your insulin is not working effectively—or if you don't produce enough of it—sugar and fat build up in your blood vessels. Insulin also causes the kidneys to retain salt. This combination results in high blood pressure (hypertension), diabetes and cardiovascular disease which can lead to heart attacks and strokes. Ultimately, this is all due to the excess fat and almost always responds to weigh reduction. As you can see, people with a BMI greater than 25 definitely can benefit from weight-reduction counseling.

Scientists have shown a relationship between high BMI and increased risk of other diseases and conditions, including:

- Cancer (particularly uterine, breast and colon cancer)
- Liver disease
- Gallbladder disease (including gallstones)
- Infertility
- Osteoarthritis
- Depression
- Sleep disorders like sleep apnea
- Gastroesophageal reflux (heartburn)

We must address obesity and its related disorders. Unfortunately, there is not a lot of time during the typical office visit to spend teaching about nutrition. Because of time constraints, many, if not most, physicians resort instead to handing out print materials for the patient to read after the visit or they refer their patients to dietitians. Since I have always had a passion for nutrition, I took a different route. While I work with dietitians, over the years I developed my own package of advice that I could explain in simple terms within the time confines of a typical office visit. I call it my *PVC Diet*. It's designed to be a simple, easy to remember eating guide and has provided my patients with a lot of success in managing their weight. As a result, many of my patients want to know more about my approach and have requested I write this book.

There are times where I do advise my patients sit down with a dietitian to obtain more detailed instructions, especially if they have diabetes. For over a decade now, I have had the pleasure to work with a fantastic dietitian, Joan Kanute, MS, RD. She has a sound knowledge of nutrition and what it takes to maintain good eating habits over the long haul. We have worked on many projects together, and I am pleased that she agreed to co-author this book.

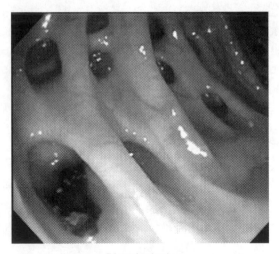

Diverticulosis

In addition to weight-reduction diets, I also commonly counsel patients on high-fiber diets. Americans do not eat enough fiber! As a result, 40 percent of us have diverticulosis—a condition where pockets form in the lining of the colon. This is probably due to most of us not being raised on a diet that contained enough fiber. Growing up in the 60s, breakfast was usually some kind of corn or rice-based cereal. Lunch was a couple of slices of white bread with one or two slices of ham or bologna. Dinner might have had meat, potatoes and vegetables, but the vegetables were often canned corn or peas. Not much fiber in this diet. The diet our children are eating today is not much better and in some ways is worse due to highly processed foods and fast foods.

I also see patients with irritable bowel syndrome, celiac disease, lactose intolerance and inflammatory bowel disease. The latter is very interesting as there are selections you can make in your food choices that will actually decrease your inflammation. Thus, I'm constantly discussing eating and nutrition with my patients.

The main topic we are going to address in this book is weight reduction through our PVC diet. I devised the PVC diet as a simple, easy-to-remember set of rules that I could explain to my patients in one sitting. Over the years, it has been very effective. With the help of Joan Kanute and my daughter, Danielle Sell, we created this book for you. I hope you will enjoy it.

I have to make one final note. As a physician, I am also a scientist. Therefore, I will at times bring in some biology and chemistry into our discussion. Don't worry, it won't be too complicated. It should actually be quite interesting and eye-opening and will help you understand the reasoning behind the PVC diet.

Through your journey with PVC, if you have any questions, feel free to reach out to us at support@pvcdiet.com or visit us at www.pvcdiet.com.

Learn the Basics

Rules of the Road

There are many diet books in print today, each designed to help people lose weight. Although they are all different and have their own individual positive points, most of them work on a single principle such as "low-fat" or "low-carbohydrate," Others expound the benefits of a balanced intake. *The PVC Diet should not be looked upon as a strict diet, but rather as a simple set of rules to assist you in choosing your food.*

We're on our own today.

In the past, food was only available based on seasonal availability and our diets automatically conformed accordingly. Today, our food industry is global and we can eat just about anything we want whenever we want. Food can be shipped to us from the southern hemisphere providing us fresh fruit and vegetables in the dead of winter. This is fantastic! We live in a wonderful era. Unfortunately, sometimes a benefit like this creates some complexities for us.

Since we have to eat multiple times every day, we frequently need to make good food decisions. This is difficult when we have the full food chain to choose from and limited time to make those choices. We also fall victim to the marketing and advertising of the food industry that is mostly interested in selling products even if they are not very healthy for us to eat.

Nutrition is complicated and therefore most of us need advice in order to make the correct food choices. The PVC diet is designed to provide you with simple, straightforward advice. There are no gimmicks or fads here, just a lot of commonsense principles rooted in scientific data.

No stressful counting plans!

The first thing you all need to know is "forget counting fat grams." They are "considered" but are not "counted" in this diet. The only thing you need to remember is PVC—three easy letters that will steer you to the correct selection of food for weight control and improved overall health.

What does PVC stand for?

PVC Diet? That must stand for the Pasta, Vino and Cheese diet that I have been known to enjoy from time to time. Actually **"P"**, "V" and "C" stand for Protein, Vegetables and Carbohydrates, three totally different food groups upon which we base this diet. It would be nice if we could live on pasta, vino and cheese though.

Every Meal Counts

Every time you sit down to eat (and if you're not sitting down, you should be), think PVC! By doing this, you will always be analyzing the nutritional value of your meal. Remember, every meal counts! We all have a bad meal here and there or indulge at a party, but it cannot become a habit or you will never lose the weight. More importantly, you can negatively affect your health.

How do we calculate our ideal weight?

How much weight do you need to lose? That depends on what you currently weigh compared to how much you should weigh. A simple rule of thumb is the following:

For a Woman:

You get 100 pounds for the first 5 feet of height + 5 pounds for each inch over 5 feet. If you are less than 5 feet then subtract 5 pounds for each inch.

Example for a woman who is 5'6" =
> First 5 feet = **100 pounds**
> 6 inches over 5 feet = 6 × 5 = **30 pounds**
> 100 pounds + 30 pounds = **130 pounds**

For a Man:

You get 106 pounds for the first 5 feet of height + 6 pounds for each inch over 5 feet.

Example for a man who is 5'10" =
> First 5 feet = **106 pounds**
> 10 inches over 5 feet = 10 × 6 = **60 pounds**
> 110 pounds + 60 pounds = **166 pounds**

This is a rough, yet simple calculation for lean body mass.

Body Mass Index (BMI)

The most commonly used method of assessing weight today is the Body Mass Index (BMI). This number is based upon the relationship of your weight to your height. The ideal BMI is 22 and is associated with the lowest chance of dying (mortality rate). Your mortality rate rises if your BMI moves in either direction. Remember, it's also dangerous to be too thin.

The figure below shows that mortality is directly related to BMI. The bottom of the "hockey stick" line is a BMI of 22. As you can see, the mortality rate rises as you depart from that point.

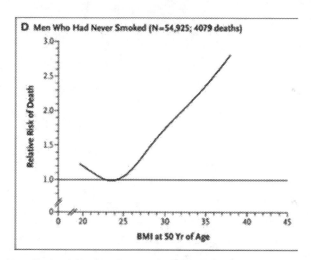

Figure: New England Journal of Medicine 2006; 355:763-778; August 24, 2006

To calculate your BMI, use the following formula:

BMI = $\dfrac{\text{Weight (lbs.)}}{\text{Height (in)}^2} \times 703$

BMI Categories:
- Underweight = less than 18.5
- Normal weight = 18.5-24.9
- Overweight = 25-29.9
- Obesity = 30 or greater

There are numerous websites that will calculate your BMI for you. You can visit ours at www.thepvcdiet.com.

If your BMI is above 25, you need to keep reading. You are at risk for serious conditions like hypertension, diabetes, heart disease, strokes and more. If your BMI is over 30 you are obese and should discuss this with your doctor as well.

How Does Your GI Tract Work?

In order for you to understand what happens to the food after you eat it, it is useful to review some anatomy and physiology of the GI tract.

The Esophagus

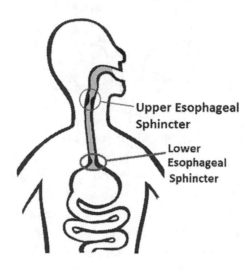

When we eat, the food first enters the mouth and then passes down our esophagus which is just a tube about a foot long that carries the food from our mouth into our stomach. It has a sphincter muscle at its entrance and another one at its exit into the stomach. These two sphincters remain constricted (like the anus) unless we are swallowing. The act of swallowing opens the upper sphincter, and the food is forced into the esophagus by the contraction of the muscles of the mouth, tongue and pharynx. The passage through our esophagus is not a passive one. The esophagus actually drives the food down through a process called "peristalsis." After all, the astronauts in the Space Shuttle can swallow just fine in zero gravity. You can swallow on your back or even if you are standing on your head. The lower sphincter then relaxes and allows the food to pass into the stomach. It then closes so that the stomach contents cannot pass back into the esophagus. If this sphincter is weak, acid reflux occurs.

The Stomach

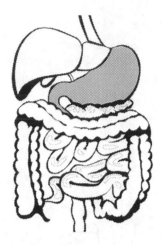

The stomach is an expandable bag that has the capacity to hold about six cups (42 ounces) at any given time. It is like an accordion, having the ability to collapse on itself or expand with the introduction of food. It is a myth that you can shrink your stomach. You really can't. You can stretch it though! In addition to its reservoir function, the stomach initiates digestion which is the process whereby food is broken down from the form in which we eat it into the basic chemicals of which it is composed. To do this, the stomach produces acid and enzymes which dissolve the food. At the same time, the stomach is very effective at grinding the food into a more simplified state that can be transferred into the small intestine, a little at a time. Thus, the stomach acts as a reservoir so we can eat at convenient times instead of having to eat constantly. It begins the digestive process and presents the food a little at a time to the small intestine where the rest of the digestive process occurs.

The other major process that is essential for us to process our food is absorption. This is the actual passage of the nutrients in their simple state across the lining of the intestine and then into the circulation system (bloodstream). This occurs in the small intestine. We have to learn about a couple of very important organs first, the duodenum and pancreas.

The Duodenum and Pancreas

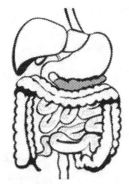

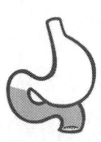

Duodenum   Pancreas

The first part of the small intestine is called the duodenum which is a C-shaped organ that receives the food from the stomach. The food coming into the duodenum is very acidic as it comes out of the stomach. The small intestine cannot handle it this way or ulcers would occur. That's why the duodenum is the most common place to develop an ulcer. To neutralize this acid, the pancreas produces sodium bicarbonate and empties its contents early into the duodenum right as the food enters before it travels on to the small intestine.

The pancreas also produces very strong enzymes, which further digest (break down) the food into its component parts: amino acids, fatty acids and simple sugars. Finally, the bile that comes from the liver is emptied into this same place which mixes with the fat in our diet to make it easier to digest and absorb. As you can see, the duodenum is a very important structure. What an ingenious design.

Digestion

Digestion is the process of breaking down food into its component parts:
- Protein is broken down into 20 different amino acids.
- Fat which is ingested as triglycerides is broken down into fatty acids and glycerol.

- Carbohydrates are broken down into simple sugars. Some of the structure of carbohydrates is not digestible. This is where fiber comes from.

The Small Intestine (SI)

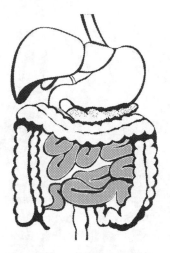

The digested food passes out of the duodenum and into the small intestine which is 18 feet long and has a "furry" lining which allows for it to absorb the digested food. The furry lining of the small intestine is due to the fact that it is like a rug with many individual folds called villi. If you flatten out the villi in your intestine, it would cover a football field. As you can imagine, it is almost impossible for us to not absorb something we eat if it is in its absorbable form. You cannot overwhelm the absorptive capacity of the small intestine. That is one main reason that obesity is so common. There is not much other structure to the small intestine. It's just a very long tube that has an incredible absorptive surface. The first half of the small intestine is called the jejunum, and the second half is called the ileum. At the end of the ileum is a specialized section where we absorb our fat-soluble vitamins like A, D, E and K. There is another sphincter here which slows down the passage of the food into the next segment, the colon.

The Large Intestine: Colon

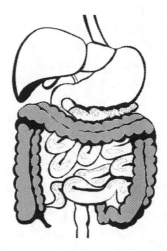

Whatever is left in the small intestine at the end of the ileum that is not absorbable (e.g.: fiber) passes into the colon in the lower right hand side of your abdomen down by your appendix. The colon is five feet long and surrounds our abdomen like a large question mark. It has two jobs, the first of which is to absorb water. About a half-gallon of water enters the colon every day. This has to be absorbed back into our bodies and the colon does this very well. The second job of the colon is to package the stool in a form that can be conveniently eliminated. We all know how important this is.

The packaging process of stool is a complex one. When our food enters the colon on the right side, the contents are very liquid. We already said that the colon absorbs about a half-gallon of water every day from the stool. This is a continuous and progressive process as the stool courses around the five-foot colon towards the left side of the body. The contents of the colon on the right side are liquid whereas they are solid on the left, which results in a different pressure situation on the right vs. the left side of the colon.

Why is this important? Well, since the colon has a low-pressure zone on the right and a high-pressure zone on the left, different things can happen to the colon as a result. The left side of the colon is where we develop diverticulosis, a condition where pockets form in the lining of the colon. These pockets are very thin-walled sacs, which can rupture. To best understand what they are, think of a bicycle tire which has an outer tire and an inner tube. Imagine you have a crack in the outer tire and a bubble of the inner tube is sticking out. This is what a diverticulum is. We want to do everything we can to decrease the pressure in the left side of our colons to avoid rupturing a diverticulum.

Fiber help avoid developing diverticuli. Eating fiber lowers the pressure in the left side of the colon. This makes diverticulosis less likely to develop and if you already have diverticulosis, it makes them less likely to rupture.

Our colons are also home to trillions of bacteria. We have them from birth and provide them a home throughout our lives. In return, these bacteria produce vitamins and other nutrients for us which they extract from the contents of our colon. Some of these can be absorbed and used as nutrition for us. There are actually more cells in the bacteria in our colons than there are in the rest of our bodies. The science of the fecal microbiome is in its infancy and is the source of much research funding today. There are over 400 different species of bacteria in humans. Each of us has his/her own mixture of them. As you will learn in a later chapter, these bacteria can also be a cause of obesity.

The Rectum

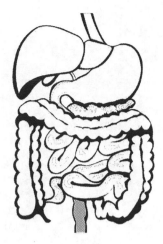

The final organ in the GI tract is the rectum, which is about four inches long and controls how we move our bowels. The rectum is very sensitive, almost with the sensitivity of the tip of your finger. It can tell if you have solid, liquid or gas in it. Imagine if you couldn't tell the difference. You would never be able to pass gas without having an accident. Needless to say, the rectum is very sensitive.

The emptying of the rectum is dependent upon its sphincter, the anus. Unfortunately, we were probably not meant to stand upright. As a result, hemorrhoids develop here in the distal rectum.

That's it, you now are experts on the GI tract. Let's use this knowledge to help us understand the PVC Diet.

How Does Your Diet Affect Your GI Tract?

We always hear about how obesity effects your heart, blood vessels and joints. Most people have no idea how much it also affects your GI tract. Let's look at how it does.

GERD

Gastroesophageal reflux disease (GERD) is a very common condition effecting almost 20 percent of the population at least to some degree. It results when the sphincter at the lower end of the esophagus fails to remain closed which allows stomach contents to bubble up into the esophagus. These contents are at times very harmful to the lining of the esophagus as they are acidic. The result is that the esophagus is burned by the acid and injury results. The esophageal lining is very similar to our skin so you can imagine what spilling acid on your skin would do.

Lower Esophageal Sphincter Closed   Lower Esophageal Sphincter Open

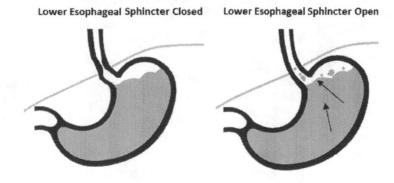

The patient with GERD usually develops heartburn when this occurs. In addition, the patient can develop symptoms that are not seemingly related to their esophagus. They can suffer with asthma, chronic cough and even sinus problems.

GERD is very definitely made worse when the patient is obese. The extra pressure that this precipitates in the abdomen increases the stress on the lower esophageal sphincter and it fails to remain closed. Obesity is definitely a risk factor for worsening GERD.

Gallbladder Disease

Obese patients are at increased risk for gallstones. We usually look upon the patients who develop gallstones as belonging to the "4F" club, they are fat, female, fertile and forty. It is very common for women who are overweight and who have had pregnancies and are middle-aged to develop gallstones. This is due to the fact that they produce bile that is saturated with cholesterol which falls out of suspension and precipitates the development of gallstones. It is estimated that 20 million Americans have gallstones and do not know they have them. About 2 percent of this population will need gallbladder surgery every year. Obesity is definitely a risk factor for gallstones.

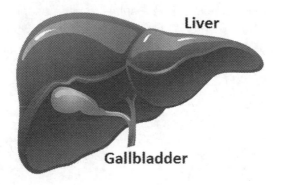

Liver

Gallbladder

Liver Disease

Obese patients are increasingly developing a disease of the liver due to excess deposition of fat. Fatty liver is today the most common cause of abnormal liver enzymes. This is due to the fact that the liver is the first organ that receives the output of the GI tract. Since it is the "chemical plant" of our body, it receives the contents of the food we eat first. Unfortunately, much of this fat never leaves the liver and deposits there. It then causes inflammation in the liver which precipitates liver injury. This injury, if allowed to continue, can proceed to the development of cirrhosis of the liver. Obesity is definitely a cause of serious liver disease.

Altered Bowel Motility
A high fat diet has an effect on how the GI tract moves. It slows it down. As a result, the stomach will empty slower. This causes it to hold on to the food for a longer period of time. If the patient then lies down or does some strenuous activity, GERD will occur.

High fat diets can slow the passage of food as it passes through the small intestine. This can result in bloating and distention. A high fat diet results in much slower colon transit. Combine this with the fact that the patient who eats a high fat diet also usually eats less fiber, and you can see that constipation will be a major problem of a high fat diet.

Altered Intestinal Bacteria
We have discussed elsewhere in this book that certain bacteria (Firmicutes) have the ability to ferment fiber into fat. This can result in as much as 500 extra calories per day as this fat is absorbed across the colon lining. So the bacteria in your colon can cause you to gain weight.
Equally interesting is the fact that patients who eat high fat diets have a higher incidence of Firmicutes in their colon. So at this time it appears that if you eat a high fat diet, you will promote the colonization of your colon with bacteria that will promote further fat intake.

As you can see, obesity greatly affects the GI tract in multiple ways. Getting weight under control is the first step to relieving the ailments described above.

Irritable Bowel Syndrome (IBS)
IBS is a condition that effects 15% of the world population and is known for its "ABCs": abdominal pain, bloating and change in bowel habits, either constipation or diarrhea. The main theories surrounding IBS include problems with altered gut motility, abnormal sensitivity and enhanced secretion. A single cause does not exist.

Bloating and flatulence (gas) are frequent complaints in patients with IBS. It has become increasingly evident that our diet can precipitate these symptoms through the interaction of the contents of our diet with the bacteria that inhabit our GI tracts.

The foods that can cause these symptoms fall into a category known as FODMAPs, which stands for: Fermentable Oligosaccharides, Disaccharides, Monosaccharides and Polyols. These substances are all sugars that are poorly absorbed in some people and cause fluid to enter the intestine. Since they are not absorbed, they pass into the colon where they are fermented by the bacteria that live there.

In order to understand how these sugars cause GI symptoms, we need to review how sugars are absorbed by the intestine. As we will discuss in the "C" chapter, carbohydrates are long chains and sheets of simple sugars connected by chemical bonds. We cannot absorb carbohydrates. They must first be "hydrolyzed" or broken down into simple sugars. Unfortunately some of us lack the enzymes necessary to break them down. Lactose is a perfect example (see "Lactose Intolerance"). There are others though who cannot break down some of the others. This leads to the movement of fluid into the intestine with its associated bloating and distention.

Even in people who can break down these carbohydrates, symptoms can still develop if they are ingested in an incorrect ratio. Table sugar (sucrose) is a disaccharide which means that it is composed of two sugar molecules connected together by a bond. The two sugars are glucose and fructose. Interestingly the cells of our small intestine can absorb sucrose very well since the transporter built into the cells that line the intestine function the best when glucose and fructose are present in equal concentrations. Unfortunately, much of our sweetened beverages are sweetened with high fructose corn syrup (HFCS). Ingestion of HFCS causes the intestinal contents to be dominated by fructose without an equal amount of glucose. This overwhelms the transporters and causes the fructose to be malabsorbed. The unabsorbed fructose then passes into the colon where it is fermented into gas by the bacteria in the colon. Symptoms therefore develop characterized by bloating, distention, gas and diarrhea.

Foods that contain the most FODMAPs include
- Apples
- Artichokes
- Asparagus
- Broccoli
- Cabbage
- Honey
- Mangos
- Onions
- Peaches
- Pears
- Peas
- Wheat and Rye
- Chickpeas
- Watermelon

P

Let's begin with some science which should help you understand how to start making good healthy decisions. The first thing you have to think of when you are deciding what to eat is the letter P.

The letter "P" stands for Protein but also refers to two other things: Preferences and Portion size.

P (Protein)

Our bodies are predominantly made of protein (P). It's what holds you together. Your muscles, bones, skin, etc. are composed predominantly of protein. In addition to being the composition of your muscles and bones, proteins are the basic structure of most of your hormones like insulin. It's the structure of your body. The major circulating protein in your body is albumin and it's unique to each of us.

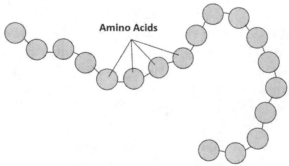

Primary Protein Structure

Proteins are usually very long molecules which are made up of strings of very essential chemicals called amino acids. There are 20 different amino acids but they all have a similar characteristic in that they contain nitrogen at one end. This is what gives them their strength. Nine of the 20 amino acids are considered "essential" in that we cannot create them and therefore must ingest them in our diet. This is a very important reason why protein in the right amount and structure must be consumed on a regular basis.

Proteins are basically long strands of amino acids of varying lengths. Interestingly, they are unique to each and every one of us. We all make slightly different proteins. This is because most of our individual DNA strands are concerned with the production of protein. Since each of us has a different DNA, each one of us has different and unique protein characteristics.

Where do we get protein? What foods contain protein? *We get protein from eating the tissue of other living things!* Therefore, to get protein, we have to eat the structure of other living things like meat, dairy products, grains and nuts. When we eat protein it is not absorbed as protein, but it is first broken down into its component amino acids. It's the amino acids that are ultimately absorbed. Therefore no matter how much protein you eat, your body must construct your proteins from scratch. Most of our circulating protein formation occurs in our livers. This is why patients with liver disease have low levels of proteins even if they eat adequate amounts.

Unfortunately, most protein sources are also fat sources and the fat they contain is often the worst kind: saturated fat. If you eat too much protein, you will therefore consume too much fat. Some of the low-carbohydrate diets actually promote too much protein intake and, along with that, too much fat. Although we are not focusing on measuring our fat grams in the PVC Diet, we are controlling our protein intake which will automatically control a major portion of our fat intake.

How much protein should a person eat in a day?
There is a formula for this based on your ideal body weight. Dietitians are very scientific about how much protein you need. They will tell you that you should eat 0.8 grams of protein for every kilogram of ideal body weight. How much is that? We already calculated our ideal weight in the last chapter (see "Learn the Basics"), but we calculated it in pounds. We first have to convert this to kilograms (1 kilogram = 2.2 pounds). To make this conversion, take your ideal body weight in pounds and divide by 2.2, then multiply by 0.8.

Here's the formula:

$$(\text{Ideal Body Weight in pounds}/2.2) \times 0.8$$

Let's apply this formula to two real-life examples keeping in mind that each ounce of protein contains 8 grams of protein:

Female - 5 ft. 3in.
- Ideal body weight is 115 pounds
- 115 lbs. divided by 2.2 pounds = 52 kilograms
- 0.8 × 52 = 42 grams of protein

Male - 5 ft. 6in.
- Ideal body weight is 166 pounds
- 166 lbs. divided by 2.2 pounds = 75 kilograms
- 0.8 × 75 = 60 grams of protein

How much meat is 42 grams (female) or 60 grams (male) of protein? We don't weigh in grams, we weigh in ounces. On the average, meat has 8 grams of protein per ounce so:

- Female = 42 grams ÷ 8 grams of protein per ounce = she needs 5.2 ounces of meat each day
- Male = 60 grams ÷ 8 grams of protein = he needs 7.5 ounces of meat each day

Hmmm . . . I don't see too many people only ordering a 5 ounce or 7 ounce piece of meat. Many people will eat a piece of meat that size or larger at both lunch and dinner. Unfortunately, they are eating excess fat in the process.

This brings up the next "P" we need to discuss, Portion.

P (Portion)
Despite what most people think, the typical American diet includes more than enough protein. In fact, most Americans are so concerned with getting enough protein that they eat far too much of it. Why is this a problem? Well, your body is pretty smart. It can convert protein into sugar

by using a process called gluconeogenesis. *If you eat more protein than your body needs, that protein-turned-sugar is eventually converted into fat. So contrary to what some other diets tell you, calories from protein are not free calories.*

PVC POINT
Calories from protein are not "free calories," only eat as much as you are supposed to eat.

In addition to the excess calories, eating too much protein can be harmful to your body. Excess protein intake places unnecessary stress on your kidneys and can injure them.

How much should you eat? We now know how many grams and ounces you need, but you can't carry a scale around with you and measure every meal, every day! Fortunately, you have a very simple measuring device right in your hand—your palm! Another "P" to remember.

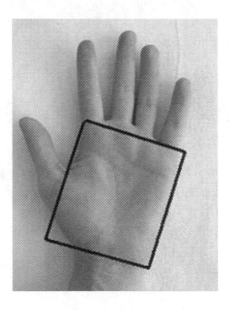

There is a longstanding recommendation by many dietitians that we should eat about a palm sized piece of meat every day. This apparently fairly closely conforms to the calculated amount of 0.8 grams per kilogram. This amount is really quite close to what you would come up with if you used a scientific calculation of grams based upon ideal body weight. The taller you are, the larger your palm. Your palm doesn't get any bigger if you're overweight though, so it's a natural, convenient and easy measuring tool!

Let's perform an experiment and see how accurate this actually is.

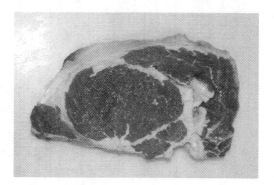

This is a picture of a typical piece of beef that you would purchase in the butcher section of your grocery store. It's also the size you would be served for a meal at most steak restaurants. It weighed 14.4 ounces. Look at all the fat in it! You can actually see it marbled in. There is much more fat in it which you can't see, though. How much of this piece of meat should you eat? Which parts of it should you cut away? The answer is in the palm of your hand.

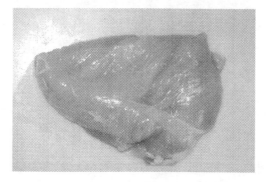

Here is another example using chicken. You can see immediately that it contains less fat. Not no fat, just less fat. This piece weighs 6.9 ounces. It's half the size of the beef. How much of this piece of meat should we eat? I've seen many restaurants which would serve this entire piece as a meal. Not uncommon to see someone eat a half chicken for a meal.

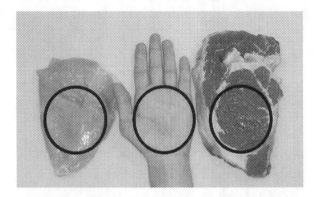

Now it's time to take out our handy measuring tool, our palm. Even though some would be inclined to eat the entire piece of meat, you really need only a small portion of it. We're going to focus on a piece of each meat source the size of the circles. How much does that weigh? How much protein does it contain?

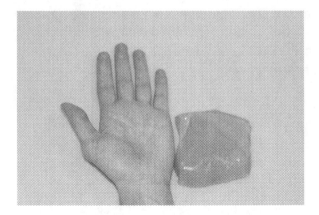

Let's cut ourselves a palm-sized piece of each of these pieces of meat for each of our two examples and see how the calculations work out.

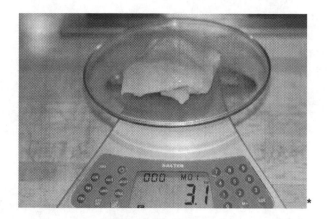

BEEF
Starting size = 14.4 oz.
Male palm-sized piece = 6 oz. or 48 gm. of protein
Female palm-sized piece = 3.5 oz. or 30 gm. protein

CHICKEN
Starting size = 6.9 oz.
Male palm-sized piece = 4.3 oz. or 36 gm. protein
Female palm-sized piece = 3.1 oz. or 25 gm. protein

In this experiment, these two palms underestimated how much protein each of these people should eat in a day. They actually needed a little over the size of their palm.

So a little over the size of your palm is the amount you need for the *entire day*. Think about the amount of protein you currently eat—you probably eat a palm-sized portion or more at both lunch and dinner. My recommendation is to focus on eating one palm-sized piece of protein per day. Most of us will eat more than this since there is protein in other food we eat and we probably split this up between two or more meals per day, which is fine, but *be conscious of the total portion for the entire day*.

PVC POINT
Focus on eating a palm sized piece of protein every day.

P (Preferences)

There are many protein sources and the amount of protein we get out of our food depends on our choice (or preference) of protein. If we eat a protein source that has a lot of fat, then we will eat more fat. If we choose more lean protein sources, our fat intake will decrease. Just overloading on protein isn't the answer though, too much can be a bad thing. Let's go into more detail on this.

PVC POINT
Few foods exist as pure sources of protein; they also contain fat and carbohydrate. You must choose wisely.

This brings up the next important component of the P: Preferences. Many factors play a role in the choice for the perfect protein source. The protein source we choose determines not only how much protein we eat, but also how much fat and carbohydrate we take in. Which proteins should we choose? Unfortunately, there are very few protein sources that are not also fat sources or carbohydrate sources. Your choice of protein is therefore very important. Remember, we are not going to count fat grams. Your fat intake will be controlled through the type of protein you consume.

The following graph lists various protein sources with their relative amounts (grams) of protein per ounce.

Grams of Protein per Ounce

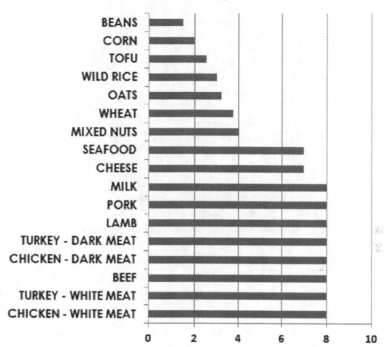

Our food selection would be easy if we could just focus on protein content, then we could choose from milk to the various types of meat with no other concern. Many people on low-carbohydrate diets follow this path. This is not always the healthiest process though.

Unfortunately, each of our protein sources is also a fat source. Take a look at this graph which compares the protein sources with their various fat contents as well.

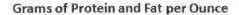

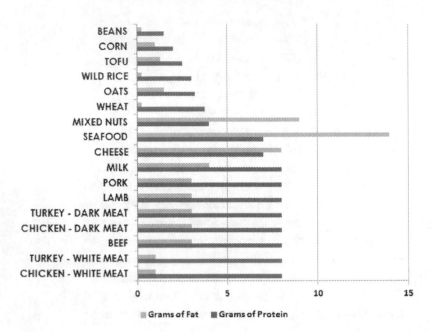

Grams of Protein and Fat per Ounce

As you can see, the amount of fat in protein sources can vary from less than 1 percent to over 50 percent. Therefore, it is important to look at not only the *amount of protein* but also the *amount of fat*. The best way to look at this is to focus on the ratio of protein-to-fat in these foods to see which ones are actually the best for you. *Your goal should be to eat the ones that give you the most protein and the least fat.*

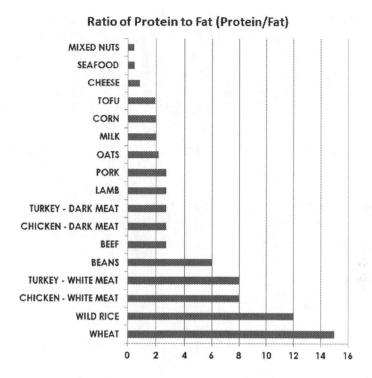

Ratio of Protein to Fat (Protein/Fat)

If we are only focusing on the ratio of protein to fat, the best source of protein would be the grains followed by white-meat chicken followed by beans. Most meat, dairy and nut choices have too much fat. You might be asking "what about fish and nuts?" Looking at the graph above, one might think fish and nuts are a poor protein choice due to their ratio of protein to fat. However, not all fat is bad for you. Some fats can actually good for you. Seafood is actually better than this table implies because the fat that is stored in fish is very good for you. Nuts have fat that is actually healthy. We will talk about this in the chapter "Good Fats vs. Bad Fats."

If grains are on one end of the spectrum, cheese is on the other. Per ounce, cheese has more fat than protein and much of it is saturated fat. You can see that cheese is not your best source of protein. Nuts are at the bottom of the table for percentage of fat, but as I said above, they are healthier than cheese since the fat they have is mostly mono-*unsaturated*. You really cannot make cholesterol out of this kind of fat, but keep in mind it's still fat though as far as calories are concerned.

Almost there, we need to consider carbohydrate content.
While just choosing low-fat protein options seems like the right strategy, we have to keep in mind that some low-fat protein sources also contain carbohydrates, which can seriously add to your caloric intake. An example is the grains which may be low in fat, but also contain 16 grams of carbohydrate per ounce. This makes using grains as a primary source of protein more difficult unless you are very physically active and can burn up that carbohydrate load (see "Why Some Vegetarians are Doughy").

Unless you are extremely physically active, you have to limit your intake of other carbohydrates when your major protein sources are from grains or beans.

The following table lists carbohydrate content to the previous list of protein sources.

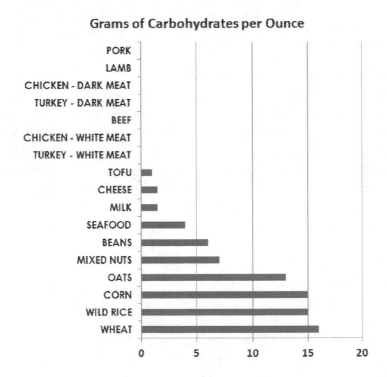

Grams of Carbohydrates per Ounce

So you see, the selection of our most healthy protein source is not a simple one. It takes some thought about protein content, fat content and carbohydrate content.

A very interesting view is all three of the components together:

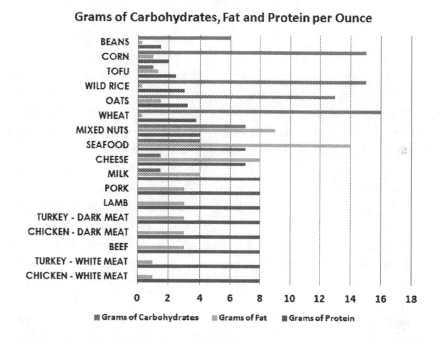

Grams of Carbohydrates, Fat and Protein per Ounce

Let's look further at our protein sources.

Meat and Eggs

Meat and eggs are predominantly protein plus fat with almost no carbohydrates. Very lean meats (white-meat chicken and white-meat turkey) are terrific protein sources with the highest ratio of protein to fat. These are 75-95 percent protein. Whole eggs are about 50 percent protein and 50 percent fat, yet egg whites are virtually 100 percent protein. The fat in egg yolks is not really unhealthy as it contains high Omega-3s (see "Good Fats vs. Bad Fats").

Fish and fowl are truly your best choices for protein. That's not to say you can't have a steak or a pork chop every now and then; they just shouldn't be the mainstay of your diet. Why do we choose these protein sources? Just think about it: a bird isn't going to get off the ground if it's too fat and a fish can't swim if it's too fat, but a pig or a cow can get very fat and still exist. When we eat these animals, we eat their fat along with their protein. In fact, marbling of fat is built into beef so that it tastes better. This is also why even white-meat pork is not as healthy as white fowl meat.

If you choose beef, you may be asking if grass-fed is better for you than corn-fed. Grass-fed beef has less fat overall (one-third to one-half less), and higher levels of beneficial Omega-3 fats. Additionally, there are higher levels of Vitamins A and E in grass-fed beef and the cows are less likely to have been given growth hormones or antibiotics. So, while grass-fed beef is better than corn-fed, white-meat fowl and wild-caught fish are still the healthiest choice of animal protein and fat.

Fish and Shellfish
Fish are interesting. Wild freshwater fish that live in the cold waters build a layer of fat on their bodies to insulate them from the cold. Since these fish are predominantly vegetarian (and not corn-fed), their fat is high in Omega-3 fatty acids. Omega-3 fatty acids promote circulation and are good for you to eat.

Shellfish and non-oily fish (flounder, haddock) are similar to lean, white-meat fowl with 75-95 percent protein content. Oily fish (salmon, swordfish) are about 50 percent protein and 50 percent fat but they are great protein choices because they contain the healthiest type of fat. I don't worry about the fat I eat from wild-caught cold-water fish like salmon and swordfish. Those little ones like sardines and anchovies are even better since they are herbivores (vegetarians) and are great sources of Omega-3s. We'll talk more about Omega-3s and the difference between farm-raised and wild-caught fish in the chapter "Good Fats vs. Bad Fats."

Dairy
Dairy products are good sources of protein, but they contain fat and carbohydrate as well. Whole milk is the basis of all dairy products, containing about 50 percent animal fat, 30 percent carbohydrate and only 20 percent protein. The carbohydrate portion is predominantly "milk

sugar" or lactose. Low-fat dairy products are made by removing the fat so the percentage of protein and carbohydrates increase. For cheese, the whey, which contains mostly carbohydrates, is removed, leaving about 25 percent protein and 75 percent fat.

Non-Dairy Milk
There are many alternatives to choose from if you don't drink cow's milk: soy, almond, rice and oat are the primary types. Let's look at their differences to help you decide which is best for you:

- Soy milk is most comparable to cow's milk in protein and the highest in protein of all the non-dairy alternatives.
- Almond milk is lower in calories and sugar, and contains the same heart healthy monounsaturated fats found in olive oil.
- Rice milk is the lowest in protein and tends to be higher in sugars and calories, yet it is non-allergenic.
- Oat milk provides moderate protein and fiber, yet is also high in sugar and calories.

Beans
Beans are mostly carbohydrate with some protein. They are an important source of protein for vegetarians. If you're using beans as a significant protein source, you'll want to significantly limit other starchy foods like breads, cereal, pasta or rice. You also will need to be very physically active to burn up the carbohydrate load.

Nuts
Nuts are another important protein source for those who avoid animal product. Unfortunately, they are, on average, 75 percent fat with 15 percent carbohydrate (starch and fiber) and 10 percent protein. The fat they contain is mostly mono-unsaturated, but proportionately, nuts are still very high in fat. Nuts are a good source of healthy fat, but should only be consumed in small amounts.

Tofu
Tofu is a great protein source for those who do not want to depend so heavily on meat. It is made from curdling soymilk and has a consistency like soft cheese but nutritionally is very different. Tofu contains all the

amino acids and is therefore considered a complete protein source. It has twice as much protein as fat. In addition to being a good protein source, it is useful as a source of plant estrogens (phytoestrogens) which is good for both women as well as men since weak estrogens decrease the incidence of cancers of the breast and prostate. Tofu comes in many different forms and consistencies and can be incorporated into many recipes in delicious ways.

Grains

Grains like wheat, corn, barley and rye are a mainstay of all diets as they are good sources of protein and are low in fat. The main issue with grains is that they contain a large amount of carbohydrate which limits their use as the main protein source unless you are very physically active. A person who exercises heavily every day or who works a physical job can use grains as their main source of protein. Most of us do not have that luxury. They are also one of our largest sources of Omega-6s and can promote inflammation. See the chapter "Good Fats vs. Bad Fats" for more details.

Vegetables

Vegetables are a great source of vitamins and minerals, but they are not a good source of protein. They do not contain enough protein by themselves to be considered a good source of high-quality protein. Vegetable protein is considered to be incomplete, which means if you eat a diet based in vegetables you are probably not getting all of the essential amino acids your body needs to function.

Putting it all together

As you can see, your choice of protein will determine not only how much protein you get, but also how much fat and carbohydrate. Therefore, your choice of protein is key to not only weight control, but also cardiovascular health. Although none of the protein sources are forbidden, the main ones that are consumed should be near the top of the list above.

We have taken all of these issues into consideration and have created a "PVC Protein Rating," which is based on the ratio of the difference between the protein content against the fat and carbohydrate content. We also added in a factor for the type of fat that the protein source contains (saturated, monounsaturated, etc.).

$$\frac{\text{Grams of Protein}}{\text{Grams of Fat + Grams of Carbohydrate}}$$

Our final rating is shown in the table below.

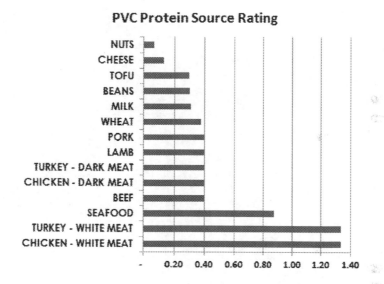

PVC Protein Source Rating

PVC POINT
Only eat protein from animals that flew or swam when they were alive.

The bottom line is to stick with fish and fowl as your protein sources. You will get the healthiest form of protein. An exception to this would be grains. This is only if you're extremely physically active, like if you are training for a triathlon. Then the grains are a very useful source of protein as you will likely burn up the carbohydrate they contain.

For the vegetarians tofu represents a major protein source. It provides twice the protein as fat and is low in carbohydrate. Always stick with low-fat tofu, though.

That's it for Protein. Now it's on to "V" for Vegetables.

V

***

"V" stands for Vegetables.

Over the centuries, human beings have been either "hunters" or "gatherers." We hunted animals and gathered what grew from the ground. Practically speaking we were omnivores, which means we had the ability to eat both meat as well as vegetables. You can tell this from our teeth. We have sharp teeth in the front of our mouths to tear meat and flatter teeth in the backs of our mouths to grind the vegetables/grains. Animals that are purely herbivores (vegetarians) like horses and cows have only grinding teeth. Animals that are carnivores (meat eaters) like cats have only the sharp teeth.

In actuality, we were much more gatherers than hunters since it wasn't always easy to find and kill an animal using primitive weaponry. It was much easier—and more predictable—to farm and harvest the bounty of the land. It's been only the last hundred years or so that we have industrialized the raising of animals to the point that we no longer need to hunt for our food. *Since human beings have been adapting much longer than 100 years, our bodies are more suited to the products of gathering rather than those of hunting.*

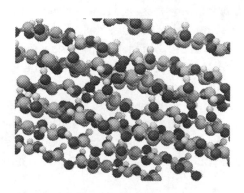

Cellulose

Over time, our bodies adapted so that we can survive on the nutrition present in plants. Plants are a great source of vitamins, minerals, and some protein. They are low in calories and create bulk which promotes healthy bowel function. Cellulous fiber is the material in the cell walls of vegetables that gives them their basic structure and strength. It is also responsible for the bulk of the protein intake of animals like cows and horses. Animals' bodies contain the proper enzymes to digest cellulose through a process called rumination. Unfortunately, our digestive systems lack the enzymes necessary to break down the cellulose fiber in vegetables. For us, much of the caloric value in vegetables are "locked in" and do not add to our calorie intake. Instead, they are passed through our small intestines and into our colons where they act as bulk agents for our bowels.

Vegetables are low in sodium and high in potassium, that's why most people prefer to salt them. From a clinical point of view, this is very important. Since humans previously existed mostly on plants, our bodies adapted. Since by existing on vegetables, we were eating large amounts of potassium and much smaller amounts of sodium, our kidneys adapted to retain sodium but lose potassium. This was essential when we were mostly gatherers eating vegetables in order to retain enough sodium and not build up too much potassium as the balance of sodium (Na) and potassium (K) must be closely regulated.

Catapult yourself to present day. Since most Americans do not eat enough vegetables, we are now consuming a diet that is very high in sodium and low in potassium. Recent studies have shown that 99 percent of U.S. adults consume more sodium daily than recommended by the American Heart Association, which recommends we ingest only 1,500 mg. The Institute of Medicine's Tolerable Upper Intake Level is (2,300 mg.). Most Americans are eating far in excess of this, many routinely ingesting over 4,000 mg. per day. This leads to high blood pressure (hypertension) and all the cardiovascular complications like heart attacks and strokes. The real problem is that hypertension is a silent illness. You really do not know if you have it as it does not cause symptoms.

We are eating excess salt because our industrialized food industry can provide us with any food at any time and wants to provide us tasty food.

In addition, more than 75 percent of sodium intake is from packaged and restaurant foods, which makes it difficult for individuals to reduce their own sodium intake. Since our taste buds mainly respond to salt, fat and sugar, the food industry has filled our diets with these to get us to eat their products. *As a result, we are eating too much sodium and not enough potassium.* The average "meat and potatoes diet" presents our kidneys with excess sodium every day and not enough potassium. As a result, hypertension (high blood pressure) is rampant. Combine this with the obesity problem, and one in three adults has hypertension today and 60 percent of diabetics suffer with it. It's a real problem.

How do we physicians treat patients with hypertension? What do we put patients on who have hypertension? We use diuretics, one of the safest and best tolerated families of medications for high blood pressure. Diuretics lower blood pressure by causing the loss of excess fluid by forcing the kidneys to eliminate sodium. They basically interfere with the kidney's ability to retain sodium. Unfortunately, these drugs also cause the kidneys to spill potassium into the urine, which can be very dangerous. Low potassium can cause heart rhythm issues and at times profound weakness. As a result of these medications and the loss of potassium they cause, patients often need potassium pills. The ironic thing is that most of these patients would not even have high blood pressure if they ate like gatherers as their ancestors did with a diet higher in vegetables. Eating like a gatherer—what a simple solution to a major health issue!

PVC POINT
Eat like a gatherer rather than a hunter; it will help you control your blood pressure.

Just like protein, it is important to make healthy vegetable choices too. When we refer to vegetables, we're talking about *most green vegetables* because they are the ones low in sugar. These include: broccoli, asparagus, brussels sprouts, green beans, kale, spinach, etc. Don't rely on the yellow or white ones like corn or potatoes which are high in sugar. Be careful with peas since they are high in carbohydrates even though they are green!

PVC POINT
Green vegetables can be consumed with almost no restriction. Go Green with vegetables!

Green vegetables are a mainstay of the PVC diet because we absorb the healthy vitamins, potassium and proteins from them, but not the "locked in" sugar and calories. So what's wrong with white and yellow vegetables? These vegetables, like potatoes and corn, are basically composed of starch which is just a long chain of sugar molecules. Starch is immediately converted into sugar in your stomach after you eat it. *Eating a potato is no different than scooping a spoonful of sugar out of your sugar bowl.* What do we do with potatoes? Since they don't have too much taste, we put salt and fat on them! So take that spoonful of sugar, add some butter and salt to it and that is what you are getting when you eat a potato.

You really don't need to limit how many green vegetables you eat in a day, but *watch how they are prepared.* This does not mean that you can cook them in butter or other oils that contain saturated fat. *Deep-frying vegetables completely negates any of the health benefits.* If you need to add a bit of fat to your veggies, make sure it's a healthy type like olive or canola oil.

Even a veggie tray can be unhealthy if you're not careful about what you dip the vegetables into. Creamy veggie dips can contain 15 grams of fat per tablespoon. Since we already told you that you have about 45 grams of fat allowed in a day, this can really add to your fat intake. Use yogurt instead.

Let's rate the vegetables.
We've created a "PVC Vegetable Rating," which is based on their vitamins, potassium and proteins in correlation to their carbohydrates.

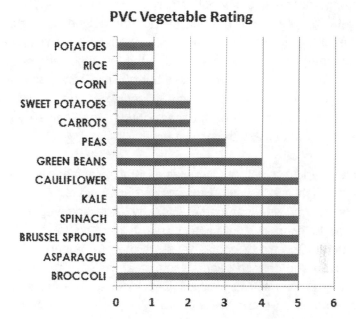

As you can see, the greener the vegetable, the better!

PVC POINT
Half the circumference of your plate should be "green."

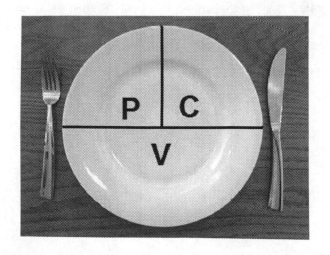

It's amazing how many of my patients, mostly men, will say, "I just can't eat vegetables. I can't stand the taste." Longstanding aversions to vegetables that were poorly prepared when you were a child, along with taste buds that have been accustomed to the fat, sugar and salt present in today's common food sources contribute to this sentiment. As I said earlier, vegetables are by nature low in sodium, sugar and fat. Since these are the main stimuli of your taste buds, vegetables need some preparing in order to make them palatable.

A favorite of mine is roasted vegetables that have been sprayed with olive oil and lightly seasoned. Brussels sprouts, asparagus and broccoli are all wonderful when prepared this way. Roasting vegetables is a terrific way to bring out delicious flavors in the vegetables and retain their nutrients. Too many people resort to the pre-prepared processed, frozen, boxed and canned vegetables instead of learning to take a few minutes to prepare fresh vegetables. Check out some sample recipes in the "Recipe" section of our website. With the wide variety of vegetables offered at local grocery stores, keeping the vegetables in your meals interesting is easy.

So, get ready to make green vegetables the mainstay of your diet. Our ancestors lived very well on them and our bodies are designed to thrive on them. There would be much less obesity, hypertension and diabetes if we all migrated to a diet that was 50 percent green vegetables.

The next letter is "C" for carbohydrates.

C

"C" stands for Carbohydrates.

Most of the food we consume is in the form of carbohydrates. These include the starches and sugars that we eat every day, all the bread, pasta, rice, potatoes, candies, cakes, cookies and sweets. Many Americans have never eaten less fat than they do today and yet they have never been fatter. *This is in part due to the fact that we eat far too many carbohydrates.*

What is even more important is the fact that there is often a large amount of fat consumed with the carbohydrates. This is because carbohydrates do not typically have much taste and, like other vegetables, they are low in sodium. So what do we do with them? We salt them and we spread fat over them. Even worse we dip them in boiling fat like French-fries and chips. This makes carbohydrates a big problem today. They are a major source of our health issues.

Believe it or not, our bodies cannot store very many carbohydrates. We really can't store more than we can use in a day. Just think about what the athletes do the night before a marathon race: they eat large amounts of carbohydrates (pasta, rice, etc.) in order to have enough energy for the race the next day. Why do they do this? *Because our bodies cannot store more carbohydrate than the energy required for about one day.*

The carbohydrate we can store is maintained in our livers in the form of a chemical called glycogen, which is designed to be rapidly converted into sugar. The liver is not capable of storing more than a small amount of glycogen. What happens to the extra carbohydrate we consume? You guessed it; it is converted into fat! *So we don't accomplish anything when we eat low fat diet foods that are mostly carbohydrate if we are consuming more than we can burn as energy the next day. It just becomes fat anyway.* This is why "C" is the last and in many ways, the most important letter in PVC. *We need to decrease the amount o carbohydrate we consume or we will never lose the weight.*

What does our body do with carbohydrates? It burns them as energy. That's the only thing we can do with carbohydrates. They are energy food, that's it. How much carbohydrate should you eat in a day? The answer is how much energy will you need and how much stored energy do you already have in your fat stores. This is the only place we are going to discuss grams. Luckily, most foods today have a clear indication of their carbohydrate content on the nutritional label (see "Let's Look at Labels"). *Ideally, you shouldn't eat more carbohydrate in a day than you will burn as energy in that day.* For the average American this comes down to about *250 grams per day.* If you want to lose weight, you must eat less than that. If you want to lose more rapidly, decrease the total carbohydrate you eat in a day down to near 100 grams. I usually tell my overweight patients to limit their carbohydrate intake to 100 grams per day and the carbohydrates you get from your green vegetables are free.

All carbohydrates are not bad though. In fact, they are some of the healthiest foods we eat! The best source of carbohydrate is fruit for several reasons:

- The sugar in fruit is easily digested and absorbed
- Vitamins are abundant in fruits
- Healthy fiber is contained in the pulp
- Antioxidants in the colorful skins protect you from heart disease and cancer

Therefore the best carbohydrates are those that come from fruit.

PVC Point
Eat colorful fruit and vegetables. The color usually means that there are high levels of antioxidants which help you avoid cancer and heart disease.

No free lunch!
As with all other food groups, there are good fruits and there are those that you should limit. The table below summarizes the grams of sugar for every 100 grams of fruit by the type of fruit.

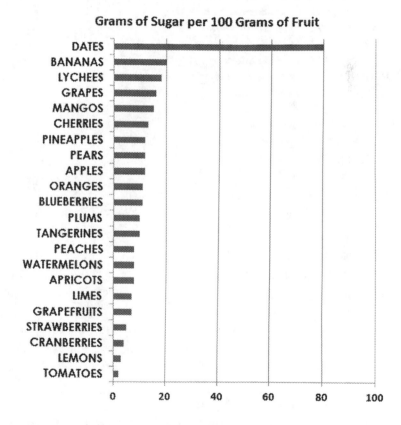

Grams of Sugar per 100 Grams of Fruit

Obviously dates really stand out for their sugar content. If we remove dates from the list, you will see the others that you should be careful of are bananas, lychees and grapes.

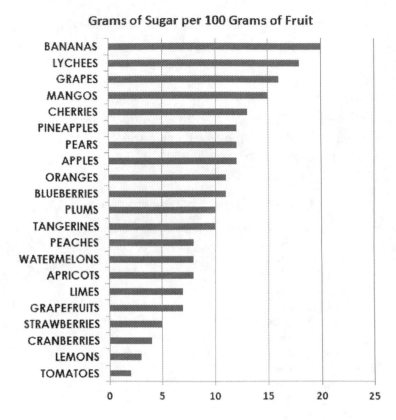

Grams of Sugar per 100 Grams of Fruit

I can't tell you how many people start their days with a banana. They think they are doing themselves good by having potassium. Instead they are starting the day with sugar (see "It's All in the Timing"). Again, there is no free lunch here. These grams of carbohydrate come out of your total for the day. Fruit is the healthiest form of carbohydrate though because of all the other beneficial components like vitamins and antioxidants. We just have to be selective about what fruit we eat.

One Potato, Two Potato
If you love potatoes, you may be wondering about sweet potatoes as a substitution for white potatoes. There is a modest nutritional advantage to choosing the sweet potato, because it has a significant difference in soluble fiber and beta-carotene content. They still should be looked at as a carbohydrate and not a vegetable.

The Glycemic Index: PVC View

While we are speaking of carbohydrates, now is a great time to share a few facts (and myths) about the "Glycemic Index." The theory behind the Glycemic Index (also known as Glycemic Load) is that all carbohydrate-containing foods can be ranked by how quickly they elevate blood sugar. The theory states that the more rapid rise in blood sugar following consumption of these foods is harmful to health and may contribute to heart disease, diabetes, cancer and obesity. One popular diet book even goes so far as to promote the Glycemic Index as the "key" to lifelong health! I'm here to tell you this is not completely true.

The main problem is the lack of standardization of methods for determining a food's Glycemic Index. Methods vary, results are inconsistent and the amounts of food tested are unlikely to be what is usually consumed. For instance, when the Glycemic Index first became popular in the early 1980s, carrots were listed as one of the highest and so the recommendation was to avoid eating carrots. The amount of carrots tested was close to 1 ½ pounds! It's unlikely that any of us would eat 1 ½ pounds of carrots in one sitting! Also, foods are tested without any other foods, and we all know that we rarely eat just one type of food at a meal. Finally, by adding a little fat to food, there is a dramatic decrease in the Glycemic Index. This would seem to be a good thing if you followed Glycemic Index alone, yet we all know it's not.

What is the bottom line for the Glycemic Index? It remains an UNPROVEN theory. The many other strategies we've outlined in the PVC diet, such as focusing on a plant based diet, are proven to be effective in promoting health.

Nutrition Facts

Nutrition Facts
Serving Size 1.25 Cup (286g)
Servings Per Container 5

Amount Per Serving

Calories 310   Calories from Fat 110

%Daily Value*

Total Fat 12g	**18**%
Saturated Fat 4g	**20**%
Trans Fat 0g	
Polyunsaturated Fat 1g	
Monounsaturated Fat 5g	
Cholesterol 20mg	7%
Sodium 290mg	12%
Potassium 780mg	22%
Total Carbohydrate 36g	12%
Dietary Fiber 12g	48%
Sugars 6g	
Protein 17g	

Vitamin A 20%	•	Vitamin C 80%
Calcium 20%	•	Iron 20%
Vitamin E 8%	•	Vitamin K 110%
Thiamin 25%	•	Riboflavin 20%

As I said above, fortunately most food items you buy today will have nutrition facts printed on the packaging. This will list the number of grams of carbohydrate. The first thing you should do is to *look at the number of servings per container and the size of a serving.* This is very important (see "Let's Look at Labels"). Then count the total grams of carbohydrate per container by multiplying the grams of carbohydrate per serving by the number of servings per container. You will be amazed at how many grams of carbohydrate you consume in a day. Remember, carbohydrates are dense and contain about 4 calories for every gram of their weight. This really adds up.

Carbohydrate Drinks

Do you drink most of your carbohydrates? Many Americans do! One of the major sources of excess carbohydrates today is in what we drink. The average soft drink has over 40 grams of carbohydrate which translates to almost 200 calories of pure sugar. *That's 10 teaspoons of sugar!* This doesn't just pertain to carbonated beverages. Anything that is sweetened is likely to contain the same load of calories. Sport drinks are an excellent example. Fruit drinks often are no better. It's amazing how many people consume most of their calories from their drinks! As a result, the City of New York has put a ban on large sweetened drinks.

Take a look at the chart below. It graphically depicts the number of teaspoons of sugar found in various drinks such as soda, juice and sports drinks. Now think about literally putting that much sugar into your mouth at one time. Yuck.

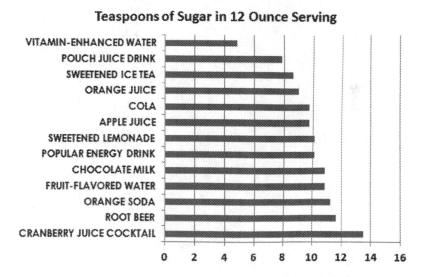

Teaspoons of Sugar in 12 Ounce Serving

An additional issue is the fact that most soft drinks in the U.S. are sweetened with high fructose corn syrup. There is a lot of debate today as to whether high fructose corn syrup is more dangerous to us than regular sugar. There are some who believe that it's responsible for the rising diabetes problem. I'm not going to comment on this as there is much debate on this topic, but will only emphasize that whether you're consuming regular cane sugar or high fructose corn syrup, the calories are the same.

The bottom line with carbohydrates is that they are only used for energy that is needed on the day that they are consumed. If you eat more carbohydrate than you can burn in a day then the excess is converted into fat. It's as simple as that. If you want to lose weight, you have to decrease your carbohydrate intake below what you are burning as energy.

THE PVC DIET SIMPLIFIED

- Focus on eating a palm sized piece of protein in an entire day from an animal that either swam or flew when it was alive.
- Calories from protein are still calories and are therefore not "free" calories.
- Beware of the fat and carbohydrate content of protein sources.
- Make sure half the circumference of your plate is filled with green vegetables—they can be consumed with almost no restriction! Cook them in a healthy manner though.
- Our bodies cannot store more carbohydrates than the energy required for about one day—the excess just turns to fat. If you are significantly overweight, you should consume no more than 100 grams of carbohydrates per day.

That's it! Not a difficult diet to remember or to stick to. There is no better time to get started than today.

There is No F in PVC

Why there is no F in PVC.

Why is this not the PVCF diet? Why aren't we concerned with fat intake? Actually we're very concerned with fat intake. The reason we aren't focusing on fat is that most of the fat we eat is actually embedded in the other "P", "V" and "C" food choices we make. We don't usually go out and eat just fat. Therefore, "F" is not a separate category in the PVC diet. People don't typically say, "I have a taste for some fat." Rather they say, "Let's have a burger," or pizza or french fries. That's how the fat gets into our diet—through the poor protein (P) and carbohydrate (C) choices we make. Don't forget, even the veggie (V) can be an unhealthy choice too if it's swimming in bad fats, heavy salt or deep-fried (e.g., fried green beans).

As you learned in the "P" chapter, it is very important we choose low-fat protein sources. The best choices are animals that either flew or swam when they were alive. That bird is not getting off the ground if it is fat and equally the fish will not be able to swim with excess fat. (They have healthy fat though. See "Good Fats vs. Bad Fats.") On the other hand, our land animals—like cows and pigs—can exist just fine with excess fat. Actually, they are bred specifically to have more fat since Americans prefer the taste. We like marbled fat and specifically choose pieces of meat that contain it.

Why does our meat contain so much fat? Much of the reason is the way we feed livestock. Although our livestock are genetically designed to live on grass, our livestock industry feeds them corn-based meal because corn is plentiful in our country. In addition, they overfeed them so that they rapidly gain weight and can be brought to market quickly. This lowers the cost of raising them. Cows are fed so much that they sometimes gain over 100 pounds per week before they're slaughtered. These animals do not have very long lives and are slaughtered quite young, so cardiovascular disease is not an issue for them. It is a significant issue for us though. When we eat their meat, we also eat their fat. It's saturated and very unhealthy.

Why do we feed them corn instead of grass? This is an economic issue. Corn grows very well in the U.S. We produce over 13 million bushels of corn per year and we consume the great majority of it. Most of our corn goes to feed our livestock. As a result, our government has been subsidizing the corn industry for many years. In addition, there are tariffs on the importation of sugar cane since it would economically hurt our corn farmers. That is why you can't find a soft drink sweetened with sugar. It's all sweetened with high fructose corn syrup.

Let's talk about how the feeding of corn to our livestock has affected them and us. Remember, whatever they eat, we eat. Most of our cows, pigs and chickens (even our farm-raised fish) are fed corn instead of the grass and seeds they were designed to eat. Unfortunately, these animals were not designed to exist on a diet made of corn. They are supposed to be eating grass—high Omega-3 healthy grass. That is the way their bodies were designed. What happens to them when we feed them corn? A lot!

I told you in the "V" chapter that cows can exist on grass because they have a special digestive process called rumination. Cows can pass their grass between two sections of their stomachs and digest cellulose. Unfortunately, when they are fed corn, their ruminating stomachs build up bacteria that produce a large amount of gas that can kill the animal. To counter this, our livestock industry feeds them antibiotics to kill the bacteria. Unfortunately, these are the same antibiotics that are used today to treat infections in humans. As a result of the use of antibiotics by the food industry, we are seeing tremendous bacterial resistance develop which makes our antibiotics less useful to us when we have an infection.

In addition to its effect on animals, corn may be the mainstay of our farming industry, but it's not the healthiest source of food for humans or livestock. Cornstalks today have been genetically designed to stand straighter. This allows the farmer to grow more cornstalks per acre and therefore increase production. Unfortunately to get cornstalks to do this means a change in their chemistry. As a result of the genetic engineering, our corn today is high in Omega-6 fatty acids. These are solid at room temperature and help cornstalks stand straighter. Unfortunately, they promote inflammation and cardiovascular disease. Grass, which is high in Omega-3s, does just the opposite of Omega-6s. They decrease inflammation and promote more healthy cardiovascular status. When we eat an animal that was raised on high levels of Omega-6 fatty acids, we alter the balance in our bodies as well. Americans are consuming far too many Omega-6s. As a result, we have a lot of arthritis and heart disease. We may be taking Omega-3 capsules, but we are eating so many Omega-6s that the effect is negated. (See "Good Fats vs. Bad Fats")

Why would our federal government subsidize an industry that ultimately makes our food unhealthy? I really have no good answer for you on this other than politics is more powerful than common sense.

Protein is not the only source of fat in our diet. Our carbohydrates are the other major source. Just look at the typical potato served at dinner. Potatoes are almost always combined with fat and salt because potatoes really have no taste otherwise. French fries, potato chips, even baked potatoes are usually smothered in butter and sour cream. Don't be fooled by the now famous sweet potato fries or even fried green beans. They are still fried.

Look at our snack foods. Sticking with potatoes, let's look at potato chips. Classic potato chips have about 10 grams of fat in every ounce (15 chips). That's almost a gram of fat per chip! Cheese puffs are very similar. There is about a gram of fat in each cheese puff! Corn chips are also the same. Basically it takes about this much fat to make carbohydrates a tasty snack. Add to this the fact that a 1-ounce portion of these snacks has 10 percent of your entire day's sodium content. These are very unhealthy snacks.

Veggies can be fat sources too. Many people dip their veggies into creamy dressings like ranch dressing. This contains 15 grams of fat for every ounce. An ounce is only two tablespoons. You can see how easy it would be to consume excess fat even when eating an otherwise healthy veggie tray.

The bottom line is that fat and its inherent health risks is imbedded into the food we eat, both naturally and after processing. In the PVC diet we focus on healthy choices of protein, vegetables and carbohydrates. If you follow the rules you just read in the "P," "V" and "C" chapters, you won't need to concern yourself with the "F." I rest my case.

Let's Look at Labels

We live in a fantastic time in a country that requires those who sell us food to tell us what's in it. They leave it up to us to decide if it is healthy though.

Most packaged food must have nutritional facts clearly and plainly posted on their labels. We've shown you one in this figure. As you can see there is a lot of information on these Nutrition Facts labels.

Nutrition Facts		
Serving Size 1.25 Cup (286g)		
Servings Per Container 5		
Amount Per Serving		
Calories 310	Calories from Fat 110	
		%Daily Value*
Total Fat 12g		**18%**
Saturated Fat 4g		**20%**
Trans Fat 0g		
Polyunsaturated Fat 1g		
Monounsaturated Fat 5g		
Cholesterol 20mg		**7%**
Sodium 290mg		**12%**
Potassium 780mg		**22%**
Total Carbohydrate 36g		**12%**
Dietary Fiber 12g		**48%**
Sugars 6g		
Protein 17g		
Vitamin A 20%	•	Vitamin C 80%
Calcium 20%	•	Iron 20%
Vitamin E 8%	•	Vitamin K 110%
Thiamin 25%	•	Riboflavin 20%

Follow these rules with Labels

Start at the top with the serving size. Each of these labels will tell you how much constitute a serving size. This is very important, since a bag of chips can have many servings. So the first thing you should do is to calculate how many servings your bag of chips contains.

The next item is the number of calories per serving, which needs to be considered in light of what your specific caloric intake is calculated to be. If this is a nonessential food item like a snack, you must make a decision as to whether it is worth eating as it may represent a sizeable portion of your total daily calories.

The next set of line items relate to the fat content. It not only provides the total fat per serving, it also breaks out the relative amounts of saturated fat and Trans Fat (see "Good Fats vs. Bad Fats"). Cholesterol is also identified. We should not consume more than 250mg of Cholesterol in a day.

Moving down, the next line item is sodium content. This indicates how much salt is contained in a serving. Table salt is Sodium Chloride. It's the sodium content that is most important though. Take a look at the example, which is for a bag of chips. There are 1485 milligrams of sodium per serving in this bag. When you consider that you are only supposed to consume about 1,500 milligrams in an entire day, you are eating almost all of your daily allotment of sodium and all of your carbohydrates in one bag of these chips. And we wonder why we're heavy and have high blood pressure.

Next you will see carbohydrates itemized. Remember, you are counting carbohydrates. These have to be subtracted from your daily amount.

Finally at the bottom you will see a line for protein. It doesn't tell you anything about the quality of the protein, just the total amount per serving. Use this to help you identify whether you are taking in adequate protein.
Make use of these labels. Always read them. They will greatly help you make good food choices. One more point. In addition to the Nutrition Facts, there will be a list of all the ingredients in the specific food choice you are considering. I have a rule. If there are more than a few

ingredients, I don't choose the item. Look for words that you understand. There are many preservatives and other supplemental items in our packaged food today. I like to keep my selections simple. The more ingredients in a label, the smaller the print. One of my other rules is if I have to put on my glasses to read the ingredients, I don't eat it.

An additional item that I like to check is the ratio of carbohydrate to protein per serving. Since we usually have to ingest about 4 times as much carbohydrate grams in a day as we do protein grams, you should try to choose foods that have about that ratio of carbohydrate to protein. Unless you are very physically active, try to maintain this ratio. The chips in the example have 7 times as much carbohydrate as protein. Not a good choice.

I have a couple of rules:

PVC Point
Don't choose food items with many ingredients—try to keep the ingredients to less than five. Also, don't choose food items with ingredients that you cannot understand. They are probably not anything you want to eat.

Good Fats vs. Bad Fats

I've spent extended time on this chapter as it is so very important to all of you. Let's start with a story.

A good friend of mine once asked me while we were eating burgers, "Which has more fat, your salmon burger or my hamburger? Which one is healthier?" My answer was that the question should not be which has more fat, but which has *better* fat.

Imagine a salmon swimming somewhere in the waters of Alaska where it is cold, very cold. The salmon has to maintain its body temperature no matter what the temperature is around it. How does it do this? It builds a layer of fat over its body that insulates it from the water temperature. The fat contained in this layer is a special kind of fat called Omega-3 that not only insulates, but at the same time dilates the arteries of the salmon. In addition, since the cold could precipitate blood clots, it inhibits the function of platelets, which are the small components of blood that promote clotting. What a great solution to a problem! The same fat that insulates the fish has special properties to open the blood vessels in that layer. Now that's engineering!

There are three major types of Omega-3 fatty acids: alpha-linolenic acid (ALA), eicosapentaenoic acid (EPA), and docosahexaenoic acid (DHA). EPA and DHA, the two most digestible, are the ones found in fish. All fish have some amount Omega-3; but fatty fish like mackerel, lake trout, sardines, albacore tuna and salmon are the best sources.

So what happens to us when we eat this salmon? We absorb the Omega-3 fat and our arteries remain open and our blood doesn't clot as fast as it would otherwise. That is why we're supposed to eat a palm-sized portion of cold water fish two or more times a week.

Fatty fish typically are cold-water fish. You have many good choices when it comes to fatty fish. The American Dietetic Association (www. eatright.org) recommends:

- Salmon
- Tuna
- Trout
- Herring
- Sardines
- Mackerel

PVC POINT
Eat a palm-sized piece of cold water fish at least twice a week to get your Omega-3s.

The above is true for *wild-caught fish only*. Many fish options at your local grocery store are farm-raised. This can be a problem. When fish are farm-raised, they are oftentimes fed corn (like our livestock) which then negates their Omega-3 advantages. Corn contains high levels of a fat called Linoleic Acid which is preferentially converted into Omega-6 fatty acids. As we said earlier, unlike Omega-3 fatty acids, Omega-6 fatty acids promote inflammation, constrict arteries and promote blood clots.

So which fat do you think is the best one to eat, the salmon or the cow? *My answer is that it all depends on how they are raised.* If the salmon is wild-caught from free water, it will have high Omega-3s. If the cow is grass-fed rather than corn-fed, it will also be higher in Omega-3s. If the salmon is farm-raised, it's probably corn-fed which negates the health benefit since it was raised on Omega-6s. This is the same for the cow. Ironically, you might be better off eating the grass-fed cow that is farm-raised than the corn-fed salmon that is farm-raised. How's that for destructive re-engineering?

Fats are necessary for us to live as our cells would not survive without them. Every one of the trillions of cells in our bodies is surrounded by a cell wall. That cell wall is composed of liquid which holds inside the water-soluble inner workings of our cells.

The most important thing to consider is the *form* of fat we are eating. It's helpful to think of the fat we eat in our diet as two separate categories: solid and liquid. The solid fat is like butter or lard. The liquid fats are the oils we consume. Let's go into some detail on this.

Solid Fat

Fat that is solid at room temperature is never good since this is how a majority of the cholesterol we eat is delivered to us.

Cholesterol

Cholesterol is a large molecule with a complicated structure. We make a lot of important hormones from cholesterol and it is intricately involved in our cardiovascular health. Even if solid fat doesn't contain cholesterol, like margarine, it still likely contains saturated fat which the body can easily convert into cholesterol. So, you see, solid fat is a major source of cholesterol or a source of the building blocks for cholesterol. Basically, don't eat solid fat—it's never good for you. What food contains solid fat? Butter, margarine and lard are the most common ones. Others include most crispy carbohydrates like chips (even baked ones) and deep fried vegetables. They are crispy because the fat they contain is solid at room temperature. Your body can convert all of this into cholesterol, so limit how much of it you eat.

PVC POINT
Don't eat solid fat.

Liquid Fat

Liquid fats are the oils. Some of them are very healthy for us whereas many of them are not. Unlike cholesterol, liquid fats are more simple chemicals that are composed of shorter chains of carbon atoms with different amounts of hydrogen attached. When the carbon atoms are "full" of hydrogen, we call them "hydrogenated." You will see this term on labels. It's not a good thing.

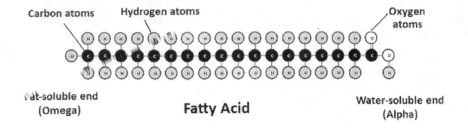

Carbon atoms   Hydrogen atoms   Oxygen atoms

Fat-soluble end   Water-soluble end
(Omega)   **Fatty Acid**   (Alpha)

The most common forms of liquid fat are called fatty acids. Basically, they are chains of carbon atoms surrounded by hydrogen atoms. The unique feature of fatty acids is that they have hydrogen at one end and oxygen at the other end which makes them "polar." This causes them to have a fat-soluble end by the hydrogen and a water-soluble end by the oxygen. We call the fat soluble end the "Omega" end and the water soluble end the "Alpha" end.

This unique feature of fatty acids makes them ideal to function as the structure of our cell walls. By lining the cell walls with fatty acids so that their fat-soluble end is on the outside and their water-soluble end is on the inside, cells can sit next to each other with their fat-soluble surfaces together and hold in their water-soluble contents inside the cell.

It's time again for some science. The photo below is a microscopic image of cells lining the intestine. They are basically lined up side by side and appear clears since they are filled with mucous.

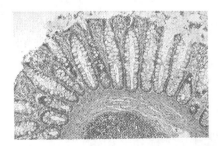

Here you see a diagram of some of these same cells. There is a lining composed of cells that are sitting side by side. One of their sides is xposed to the intestinal contents and the other is at their base.

Intestinal Contents

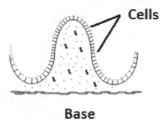

Base

If we zoom in on a single row of them they appear as you see below.

Cell Membrane

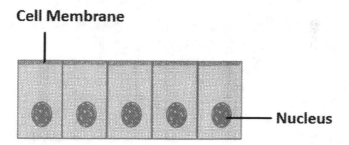

Nucleus

Each cell has a dark nucleus where its DNA is located and a thick cell membrane where it meets the intestinal contents. This is the side where absorption occurs and so the cell membrane has to be able to hold in the contents of the cell but let nutrients through and expel waste.

The cell wall is composed of fatty acids which are lined up back to back with their water soluble polar ends on the outside and their fat soluble ends on the inside.

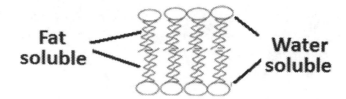

Fat soluble   **Water soluble**

This is how all our cells are formed. The walls are composed of layers of fat. Cells are not static structures though. Nutrients need to get in, and waste and carbon dioxide need to get out. Therefore, the contents of the cell wall become very important for our health. Some fatty acids promote good cell wall transmission and others do not.

The reason for the difference in fatty acids is that some of them have special bonds at different spots which alter their shape and affects their function. The one at the third carbon from the omega end and the one at the sixth carbon are really important as you will see below.

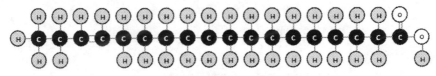

Omega-3 Fatty Acid

The Omega-3 fatty acids have a double bond at the third carbon from the Omega end. As a result of the shape that this imposes on them, they promote more rapid transfer across the cell walls. This is important in tissues like the brain where we want rapid transfer of information. The heart benefits as well since Omega-3 fatty acids stabilize cell membranes which in turn stabilizes the heart rhythm.

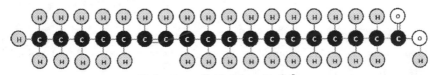

Omega-6 Fatty Acid

Omega-6 fatty acids have a double bond at the sixth carbon from the omega end. They slow transmission, just the opposite of Omega-3s. You therefore want more Omega-3s in your diet. They promote better brain function and more energy.

The table below lists the most common oils we use every day. As you can see, the ratio is radically different. All oils have more Omega-6 than

Omega-3, but some like cottonseed oil are almost 100 percent Omega-6. The best is canola oil with the lowest ratio of 2:1. This means that one-third of the oil in canola oil is Omega-3.

Fat	Ratio of Omega-6/Omega-3	PVC Rating
Flaxseed Oil	0.2:1	*****
Linseed Oil	0.2:1	*****
Canola Oil	2:1	*****
Walnut Oil	5:1	****
Soybean Oil	7:1	****
Butter	9:1	*
Lard	10:1	*
Olive Oil*	12:1	*****
Corn Oil	46:1	**
Palm Kernel Oil	46:1	*
Sesame Oil	137:1	*
Cottonseed Oil	259:1	*

The major exception on this list is olive oil. It would appear to not be one of the best oils, but actually the amount of Omega-6 oil is very low in olive oil. Most of its oil content is from monounsaturated oil which is extremely healthy for us and is the basis for the Mediterranean Diet which is very healthy.

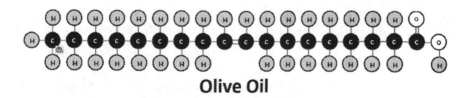

Olive Oil

The oils derived from flaxseed are extremely high in Omega-3s. The ratio in flaxseed oil is around 0.2:1 which means that it is mostly Omega-3. We should try to bring flaxseed into our diets on a regular basis.

In addition to their effect on blood vessels, one of the other major issues surrounding good fats and bad fats has to do with their effects on our levels of inflammation. Omega-3 and Omega-6 fatty acids can affect the amount of inflammation that is occurring in our bodies. This is important for arthritis and other inflammatory conditions we face. Omega-3s decrease inflammation whereas Omega-6s promote it.

It is becoming increasingly apparent that cardiovascular disease is an inflammatory process. The fatty deposits that develop in the arteries of people with cardiovascular disease have inflammatory cells within them. Therefore, the control of inflammation is critical. Omega-3s can greatly help here since they decrease inflammation.

Unfortunately, most of the fat we ingest in our diets is composed of Omega-6 fatty acids. These come into our bodies in the meat we eat, the snacks we eat and the oils we cook with. *Always look at labels—choose your fats wisely!*

Trans-fats
A discussion about fats would not be complete without a word on trans-fats. We hear a lot about them in advertising, and it is important for you to understand why they are bad and where we find them.

Trans-fats are those whose shape has been modified by the food processing industry in order to create crispness and act as a preservative. They are very harmful to us. A common way in which they are formed is when they are "hydrogenated," which means that they add hydrogen to the fatty acids and break all the double bonds. You don't have to fully understand what that word means, just that it's not healthy. Hydrogenated oils are "saturated" with hydrogen and can be very harmful to us.

PVC Point
Stay away from anything that has the words "partially hydrogenated" in it. Cook only with olive oil or canola oil.

Also, don't boil food in oil or use extreme heat with oils as you will then create your own hydrogenated oils. Even if you start with a healthy oil (e.g.: extra virgin olive oil), excessively heating it can destroy its benefits. If you are going to cook with olive oil, use the standard olive oil rather than extra virgin. Its flash point is higher and you won't destroy it as easily. Use extra virgin olive oil on your salads. Don't cook with it.

The Case for Fiber

Fiber, fiber, fiber—all we hear about is fiber. What is fiber anyway and why is it so important? How do we make sure we're eating enough fiber?

Fiber is basically the structure of plant material. Due to its complex structure, fiber passes right through our small intestine without being digested or absorbed. The most common forms of fiber come from green vegetables and whole grains. Typically, vegetables that grow above the ground like wheat, corn and oats have more fiber than vegetables that grow below the ground like potatoes and rice. After all, they have to stand up. This requires structure. Since the walls of fiber contain complex structures like cellulose that evade enzymatic digestion, fiber passes right through the small intestine intact and then enters the colon for elimination.

The colon functions much better if it contains a healthy amount of fiber. There is less spasm in the walls of the colon and things pass through much easier. As a result, there is much less constipation and less diverticulosis. We also develop fewer colon polyps if we have a healthy intake of fiber.

Once in the colon, fiber comes in contact with the trillions of bacteria that inhabit it. Some of us have bacteria (Firmicutes) that have the ability to digest some of this fiber. Unfortunately, the bacteria digest the fiber into fatty acids that can then be absorbed through the wall of the colon and into the circulation. This is another potential cause of weight gain. *Some patients actually can gain weight by consuming too much fiber.* Most of us cannot do this though and fiber is very healthy for us as a result.

PVC POINT
Fiber is not calorie-free. It can be a significant source of calories.

All fiber sources are not the same. They can be divided into two categories: soluble and insoluble. The can also be divided on the basis of fermentability by bacteria. Soluble fiber is more likely to be fermentable, whereas insoluble is most likely not fermentable. Therefore even though all forms of fiber are nutritionally good for you, soluble fiber tends to interact with the bacteria in your colon more whereas insoluble fiber does not. Soluble fiber can also lower your cholesterol, whereas insoluble fiber less so. It is mostly a bulk agent and assists you with your bowels.

So from a health point of view, soluble fiber wins out and is better for you. If you are just looking to improve your bowels, insoluble fiber may be preferable since it is less gassy. What are the sources of soluble and insoluble fiber? I've listed them below. You will note that some items exist in both categories.

Soluble fiber sources
- Legumes (beans and peas)
- Oats
- Rye
- Barley
- Fruits: prunes, plums, berries, bananas, and the insides of apples and pears
- Vegetables such as broccoli
- Root vegetables such as sweet potatoes and onions
- Psyllium
- Flax seeds
- Nuts, with almonds being the highest in dietary fiber

Insoluble fiber sources
- Whole grain foods
- Wheat and corn bran
- Legumes such as beans and peas
- Nuts and seeds
- Potato skins
- Vegetables such as green beans, cauliflower, zucchini
- Some fruits including avocado and unripe bananas
- The skins of some fruits, including kiwifruit and tomatoes

PVC POINT
All fiber is not equal.

If you are trying to lose weight, then the best form of fiber to eat comes from green vegetables! Another reason why "V" is the mainstay of the PVC diet! Veggies have much fewer calories than whole grains. Remember, if you're trying to lose weight, use green vegetables as your major source of fiber rather than whole grains.

How much fiber is the right amount?
This is a common question I am asked. My patients all want to know how many grams of fiber to eat. I usually tell them to forget the grams and look at their stool. (I can't believe how many people don't do this).

If you are passing large formed stools, then you are probably eating enough fiber. If instead you are passing skinny narrow stools or ribbons and balls (scyballous stools), then you are not eating enough fiber and need to increase it. Remember, diverticulosis is a common problem in people who do not ingest enough fiber. You can avoid getting them by starting early and eating fiber every day.

Lactose Intolerance

Lactose Intolerance is a very common condition affecting most of us if we live long enough. There are a couple of different types of lactose intolerance. There is primary lactose intolerance which occurs at birth and is relatively rare. Much more common is secondary lactose intolerance which can be a product of the aging process or can follow an intestinal infection or other condition that affects the small intestine.

Milk contains lactose which is a sugar. Lactose intolerance results when you cannot digest or absorb lactose. Like table sugar, lactose is a disaccharide which means it is two sugar molecules connected together. Unlike table sugar, lactose contains different simple sugars which are connected by a bond that requires a special enzyme to break. This enzyme is called lactase. Lactase is absent in people who have primary lactose intolerance and is either absent or decreased in people with secondary lactose intolerance.

What happens as a result? The lactose that is ingested is not broken down into simple sugars. Since it cannot be absorbed as a disaccharide, it remains in the small intestine and forces water to remain in the intestine. This creates distention (bloating), discomfort and rumbling noises in your gut. When the lactose and its fluid reach the colon, they cause more problems. The colon is not able to absorb the fluid so diarrhea results. Also, the bacteria in the colon ferment some of the lactose into gas, either hydrogen or methane. Although the hydrogen is relatively harmless, the methane can slow the motility of the colon which makes you even more uncomfortable.

The simple solution to lactose intolerance is to recognize when you have it and not eat any food that contains lactose, which includes: milk, soft cheese, ice cream, sherbet and ice milk. Hard, aged cheeses like Parmesan have very little lactose. Alternatively, you can drink one of the commercially available lactose-free milks or take lactase enzyme tablets (such as Lactaid) before consuming items with lactose. These will allow you to enjoy your dairy products without symptoms.

Since we are talking about healthy nutrition here, remember that items with lactose are typically high in fat and need to be consumed in moderation. Steer clear of full-fat cheese and whole milk*. Be careful of fat-free dairy products as they contain sugar to replace the taste removed when the fat was removed. Excess sugar turns into fat so you're not doing yourself any favors.

*Except in children under two years of age. Always speak to your pediatrician before changing your child's diet.

The Problem with Insulin

Insulin is a hormone produced by our pancreas and is most commonly associated in discussions about diabetes. We produce insulin whenever we eat sugar or carbohydrates that can be converted into sugar. Its main function is to move nutrients, predominantly sugar, out of the bloodstream and into the cells where it can be used for energy.

I like to explain insulin's role as the one who puts all your groceries away in the kitchen cabinets and closes all the doors. That is how I view the function of insulin—it takes what we eat and moves it into the cells and out of the bloodstream. Once in the cells, the nutrients can be used for our needs.

The kitchen cabinet analogy comes from the fact that insulin is a *storage hormone*, more concerned with cleaning up the counters and getting the groceries out of sight. It wants to keep them stored and not let them out. I love this description!

This is very important with respect to fat because insulin activates a hormone called lipoprotein lipase that basically keeps your fat stored. Therefore, high insulin levels make it difficult for you to burn your fat. Insulin does a couple of other important (but not so good for you) things. It stimulates appetite. Since insulin secretion peaks about two hours after we eat, we just get hungry again if we ate a predominantly carbohydrate meal.

Many people find themselves constantly hungry because they go through their day eating carbohydrates and simple sugars and therefore are constantly stimulating insulin which keeps their appetite working all the time.

The other not-so-great action of insulin is to retain salt and therefore fluid. Insulin stimulates the kidneys to retain sodium. Along with the sodium, fluid is retained. This is one of the main reasons why obese people are also hypertensive.

So you see, if you eat a diet that is high in carbohydrates, you will be producing more insulin which will cause you to:

- Store more of your nutrients as fat
- Become hungry sooner
- Retain salt and water

Following the PVC diet plan will not over-stimulate our body's production of insulin. Our goal has to be to drive those insulin levels down. Then you can release the fat stores and burn the calories.

It's All in the Timing

With what you now know about insulin, you can now understand one of the basic rules of the PVC Diet—*push your carbs later in the day!* The longer you can go without significantly stimulating insulin, the less of an appetite you will have.

So many people start their day with carbohydrates in the form of bagels, cereal, waffles, pancakes, granola, toast, smoothies and yogurt. They are setting themselves up for problems controlling their appetites, because they are stimulating insulin early in the day. They eat breakfast and then two hours later are hungry again. It's about that time that they hit the vending machines or have a sugar-containing drink or even raid the leftover donuts in the break room. Then they roll into lunch hungry again only to feed their insulin with more carbohydrates in the form of a sandwich and a few chips and cookies. Usually two hours later, they are tired in the mid-afternoon and resort to another carbohydrate pick-me-up in the form of a cookie or again hitting the leftovers in the break room. Exhausted from a long day of work (and carbohydrates), they eat their dinners (which usually contain more carbohydrates) and collapse on the couch to watch TV. Does this sound familiar?

The PVC Diet solution is to push the carbohydrates later in the day. Don't have that starchy, sugary breakfast—start your day off with a sensible breakfast of protein and only a little bit of carbohydrates. I like to have an egg-substitute omelet and maybe one slice of whole-wheat toast. On alternative days, you can have some oatmeal (with few, non-sugary toppings) which has carbohydrates but they are of low glycemic index and do not stimulate insulin as much.

Why is this so important? One of the physiologic functions of insulin is that it stimulates appetite. Since insulin levels peak about two hours after a meal that contains carbohydrates, so does your appetite. You then crave the same thing that stimulated the insulin in the first place, carbohydrates. I can't tell you how many people go through their day craving carbohydrates every two hours. It's all about fluctuating insulin levels. Our goal has to be to have low insulin levels.

Do an experiment. One day have a healthy breakfast of just an egg substitute omelet and then check to see how long it takes for you to feel hungry. On the next day have a large meal like pancakes that contains carbohydrates. Check when you become hungry after this meal. I would bet that even though the high carbohydrate meal has more calories, you will be hungry sooner after pancakes than you will after the egg substitute. I routinely have an egg substitute breakfast and do not become hungry until lunch, saving that mid-morning urge to snack.

To maintain low insulin levels, limit your lunch to a salad (for me, without meat). You will find you are not hungry until dinner. Since it's now later in the day, you can go ahead and let yourself have carbohydrates.

PVC Point
Push your carbohydrate intake to later in the day and you will postpone that rush of insulin which stimulates your appetite and starts you on your eating course for the day.

High Density and Low Density Foods

Another important tool I teach my patients is to focus on food density, which is basically the *number of calories per gram of food.* Carbohydrates, protein and fat all have different densities:

- Protein = 4.5 calories per gram
- Carbohydrate = 4.5 calories per gram
- Fat = 9 calories per gram

Since fat is a storage form of energy, it is denser than protein or carbohydrate and has twice as many calories per gram. This is very important in the food we choose on a daily basis. Let me give you some examples.

Pretzels
So many patients of mine have told me they snack on pretzels. This is understandable since they are marketed, and often recommended by health professionals, as low-fat snacks. Unfortunately, they are very dense calories since the water has been taken out and they are essentially dry calories. You can pack away a lot of calories in a small time with pretzels and not eat any fat at all. Combine this with the fact that they are so heavy in salt, and you can see why they are not on the PVC diet. Pretzels are considered a high density food. They contain over 4 calories per gram.

Cheese Puffs
Cheese puffs are one of the worst foods that you can ingest. Are you really surprised? Take a look at the nutritional information. According to one of the most popular brands on the market, almost 50 percent of their weight is fat. They are light in weight, yes, but they are very dense with respect to calories per gram.

Fruit
Fruit is just the opposite. Most of the weight of fruit is from the water contained within them. Yes, they contain carbohydrate, but this is

balanced by the fact that the great majority of weight from fruit is from the water contained within them. This brings their density down significantly, usually below 2 calories per gram. Fruit are low density foods.

As you can see, weight doesn't necessarily determine a foods density. It's a little more complicated than that. The Mayo Clinic website raises a great example of the difference between the food density of grapes and raisins. Where grapes have a very low density with 104 calories per cup, the same fruit in the form of a raisin raises the density to 434 calories per cup.

Always remember to think of food density in your choices. Look for foods that contain less than 4 calories per gram. You will be able to eat more volume of food if you choose this way.

One more point! The satiety factor of our stomach, which is what turns off our hunger, responds closely to the weight of the food we eat. Wouldn't you rather eat something of low-density that will fill you up without giving you excess calories? Makes sense to me.

PVC Point
Focus on food density. Eat foods that have a food density less than 4.

Eating in Restaurants

Don't eat the prison food!

One of the most common situations I hear from patients is they don't cook and have to eat out at restaurants most of the time, often in fast food facilities. They blame this for their weight problems. As someone who eats out at least three days a week, I have to tell you this is not the case. Follow these rules with restaurants and you will not gain weight:

- Choose only restaurants that have a "full menu" and a real kitchen. This means that "grills" are not acceptable. You can read most menus online. Make sure they have "green" alternatives like substituting a salad or side of vegetables for potatoes or rice.

- *Don't eat the prison food!* Every restaurant wants to put something in front of you while they take their time to assign staff and fill your order. What you usually receive is a loaf of bread and water. You can have the water but just not the bread! Immediately upon sitting down tell them to spare the bread and instead ask for a small dinner salad with the dressing on the side. Most restaurants have these made up in advance and can accommodate you quickly. This will give them the time they need and will give you something to eat right away. It's a win-win.

- Try eating an appetizer as your main meal. Everything is bigger today and the size of an appetizer is just about equal to what a full meal was years ago. As long as the appetizer is prepared healthy, it's a good idea to eat this as a meal. Unfortunately, many appetizers are quickly prepared fried foods so be careful with what you choose. You can make healthy foods unhealthy by frying them.

- Don't hesitate to share an entrée with others dining with you. Each of you can have a salad and then share an entrée. You will both feel full without consuming as many calories. It works. The few dollars a restaurant may charge as a sharing fee is minimal considering you're only ordering a single entrée.

- Ask your server if they offer half-portions.

- Stay away from the alcohol. You don't need the extra calories from that glass of wine or beer. Remember, one glass leads to two and along with that comes the poor food decisions that alcohol can precipitate.

- Skip the potatoes and ask for extra vegetables. Potatoes and vegetables are fairly similar in cost to the restaurant, and they usually do not care which one you want. Tell them to skip the potatoes and give you more vegetables. You don't need the carbohydrates from the potatoes or fat from the toppings/method of preparation if you are trying to lose weight.

- Remember there are calories in sauces and dressings. Don't hesitate to ask them to put these on the side so you can control how much you use.

- Dessert is not necessary but a nice thing to have. Choose a piece of fruit instead. It takes time for some of us to reach the full feeling (satiety). Resist the dessert-urge. It will go away by the time you get home.

Why Some Vegetarians are "Doughy"

It's all about the math.

Many of my patients tell me they do not eat meat. Although they are very proud of this accomplishment, most of them are overweight and don't understand why they cannot lose weight. There is a very scientific reason for this. It's their choice of protein source that is in part causing them to be overweight.

An example will help to explain. Recently, I watched a documentary on TV that told the story of a middle-aged man who gave up his previous unhealthy diet and became vegan. In addition, he embarked on a high intensity exercise program. He even became a triathlete. The man was the picture of health with almost zero body fat. His diet consisted of grains, vegetables and fruit. This is a good example of a person who is eating the correct ratio of protein to carbohydrate for his activity level. He was only able to do this because of his tremendous exercising.

Although he is eating a lot of carbohydrates, he is effectively burning them up. Accordingly, because he is so athletic and burns so many calories, he has no problem existing on grains and nuts for his protein source. We discussed earlier that these healthy protein sources are also significant carbohydrate sources. They have a high ratio of carbohydrate to protein. Unless you burn these calories, you will gain weight on this diet.

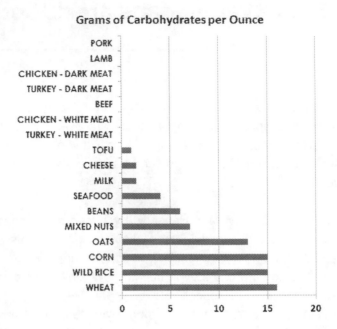

Grams of Carbohydrates per Ounce

If you are using meat as your protein source, you are not consuming any carbohydrates when you eat your protein. Alternatively, if you're using non-meat protein sources, you are almost certainly eating carbohydrate with your protein. You may be eating twice as many grams of carbohydrate than you are protein. This must be taken into consideration in calculating your total carbohydrate intake for a day. I told you earlier to try to keep your ratio of carbohydrate to protein at 4 to one or less. You can only increase this ratio if you are very physically active.

The typical patient of mine who has gone vegetarian is not nearly as active as this triathlete. Actually, most are relatively sedentary. As a result, they gain weight due to the excess amount of carbohydrates they are ingesting in their protein sources. Worse are those who use dairy products as their source of protein in addition to carbohydrate, as they ingest a large amount of saturated fat.

Meat eaters consume protein sources that contain no carbohydrate. It is easier to keep your weight down though. We've already discussed how unhealthy a diet like this can be though. The typical meat and potatoes diet is high in fat and low in fiber.

The bottom line is: if you are going to be vegetarian, you have to be very conscious of how many grams of carbohydrate you are ingesting in the process of eating protein. Remember, none of the vegetarian protein sources is free of carbohydrate. Physical activity is critical. If you are very physically active, you will have an easier time being vegetarian. You can choose grains as a protein source and still maintain your weight. If you are sedentary or only minimally physically active, then you will have some difficulty and will have to utilize other items like tofu as a protein source. You will also not be able to eat as many carbohydrates as side dishes. You will need to combine your grains with greens rather than with carbohydrates.

Follow these rules if you are at your ideal weight:

- Sedentary: 100 to 150 grams of carbohydrate per day
- Moderately active: 200 grams of carbohydrate per day
- Very physically active: > 300 grams of carbohydrate per day
- Keep your food choices around 4 grams of carbohydrate per gram of protein.
- Exercise, exercise, exercise and then do a little more exercise

Why "Natural" Doesn't Always Mean "Healthy"

Natural foods. Sounds good doesn't it? Most of the time it is, but it is getting harder and harder to find truly natural foods. At your local grocery store, the natural foods are usually those located on the edges and back of the store. You should spend most of your time in these aisles where the fruit, vegetables, poultry, fish and meat are sold. The aisles in the center of the grocery store are predominantly processed, meaning that a company took a natural food and converted it into a different product.

Not everything that is natural is healthy though for the overweight person. Remember some of the things we have told you earlier:

- Protein: be careful of your protein sources. These are all natural, but not necessarily healthy:
    - o Dairy products are high in saturated fat. Use low fat dairy products.
    - o Most livestock are fed corn today. This makes them higher in fat, specifically Omega-6s.
    - o Nuts are certainly natural, but they are very high in fat.

- Fruit: I love fruit. It is so naturally good for you. Unfortunately, it is full of carbohydrates. You don't have carte blanche to eat as much fruit as you want.
    - o Fruit counts against your carbohydrate limits.
    - o Beware of fruit drinks. They are often heavily sweetened. It may say "naturally sweetened," regardless, these calories count.

- Grains: These are a very good source of protein, vitamins and minerals, but they contain a large amount of carbohydrate. Again, watch the carbohydrate grams. There is no free lunch here. Grains have higher ratios of carbohydrate to protein than is ideal. Also, you may be one of those people who have bacteria that can ferment fiber into fat. If you become gassy with ingestion of grains, that may be you. Stick to insoluble fiber if you become gassy with grains. It will help to keep you from gaining weight.

PVC for the Aging Population

As someone who has been in practice for over 25 years, I have many elderly patients. They have aged with me over the years and many times I actually learn from them rather than them learning from me. Most of my patients in their 80s do not overeat and are not overweight. My guess is that those who did are not here anymore. I usually don't have to give eating advice to an 80 year old.

What I've learned from my "ladies in their 80s" is to eat small portions and then you can eat just about everything. Your body does not need as many calories as you age since your body mass declines, and your activity level is much lower. You must adjust accordingly or you will gain weight. If you are over 60, you've probably experienced this!

As we age, the most common suggestion I have is to eat slower and to increase vegetables and salads. Most of the older patients have gastrointestinal tracts that process food more slowly than when they were younger. The esophagus does not function as it did and therefore bites and swallows should be smaller and accompanied by more liquid. The colon doesn't function like it did in earlier years and so it needs more fiber.

Fiber is essential because most of the patients in this age group also have diverticular disease. Fiber supplementation will promote more normal colon function. Incontinence of stool can also be a problem in the elderly. This responds to fiber as well in at least 50 percent of the patients.

I usually don't have to tell an 80 year old how to eat, most of the time I learn from them.

My elderly patients have three things in common:

1. They weren't always well behaved. Most of them had the usual habits that many of us have today. They drank, smoked, stayed out, overate, etc. The key differentiating factor in this group—they knew when to stop. Most of them smile about their early days but they all knew when to say when to the bad habits.

2. They were never obese. None of my patients in their 80s and 90s are obese. I suspect they never were or else they would not be here today.

3. They remained engaged with life. Many of them still work. I've always been impressed with the drive and passion of this group of patients. They didn't retire and stop moving. A body in motion needs to stay in motion.

As I said, I get more out of them than they get out of me.

The Myth of Gluten-free

With many celebrities recently touting its health and detox benefits, you may have heard or read about the gluten-free diet and wondered if it's a good choice for you. First, if you think you have gluten-sensitivity, you should get tested by a doctor for celiac disease, an autoimmune digestive disorder. If you don't have a gluten-sensitivity, there's nothing inherently healthier about a gluten-free diet. A gluten-free diet can be healthy or unhealthy—it all depends on your food choices.

A little over 1 percent of the population have a condition called celiac disease and as a result cannot ingest a component of wheat called gluten. If they do, an immunological reaction develops in their small intestine which causes injury and malabsorption. This results in diarrhea and weight loss. Once diagnosed, treatment consists of restriction of gluten by eliminating wheat products form the diet.

A second group of patients who improve on a gluten-free diet do not have celiac disease but rather have irritable bowel syndrome. The reason they improve on a gluten-free diet is that the bacteria that live in their colons ferments wheat fiber into gas. Eliminating wheat eliminates the food for these bacteria, and the patients feel better.

If you are one of these two groups of patients, you are eliminating a very healthy component of your diet, wheat. Although this in itself is not unhealthy, what you replace it with may be. Corn products are well tolerated by those who are trying to be gluten-free. As a result many migrate to them. Unfortunately, as we said earlier, corn can be pro-inflammatory from its high concentration of linoleic acid. You would be much smarter to replace your wheat with green vegetables.

Also, some manufacturers add extra sugar or fat to gluten-free foods to improve flavor or texture, making the products very unhealthy. Gluten-free products aren't routinely fortified with iron, vitamin D and vitamin B that are in gluten-containing grain products. To follow a healthy gluten-free diet, choose naturally gluten-free grains like brown rice, quinoa and buckwheat, rather than just buying prepackaged products labeled "gluten-free." Remember, these items are still carbohydrates and still need to be eaten in moderation.

Summary

Well that's it. I've tried to provide you with useful tips and rules that are designed to help you lose weight and more importantly keep it off. This guide provides you simple rules designed to help you make healthy food choices. The best way to summarize what we have tried to teach you is to go over our PVC Points:

1. Few foods exist as pure sources of protein. They also contain fat. You must choose wisely. Choose low fat protein sources. Also be aware of your activity level. If you are not very physically active you also need to focus on the amount of carbohydrate in your protein sources. Keep your carbohydrate to protein ratio at 4:1 or less.

2. Only eat protein from animals that flew or swam when they were alive. Stay away from the land animals and certainly do not rely on dairy products. They all contain saturated fat.

3. Calories from protein are not "free calories," they contain fat and can be converted into carbohydrate.

4. The total amount of protein that you should consume every day is about the size and thickness of one of your palms.

5. Eat like a gatherer rather than a hunter.

6. Go green with vegetables! I can't emphasize more how important this is.

7. Half the circumference of your plate should be green, not white!

8. Eat colorful fruit and vegetables. The color usually means there are high levels of antioxidants which are good for you. They help you avoid cancer and heart disease. They will keep you young.

9. Don't choose food items with many ingredients. Try to keep the ingredients to less than five. Also, don't choose food items with ingredients you cannot understand. They are probably not anything you want to eat.

10. Eat a palm-sized piece of cold water fish at least twice a week to get your Omega-3s.

11. Don't eat solid fat. It does nothing good for you.

12. Stay away from anything that has the words "partially hydrogenated" in it. Cook only with olive oil or canola oil. Beware of Trans Fats.

13. Fiber is not calorie free. It can be a significant source of calories.

14. All fiber is not equal. Some of it is high in calories. Stick with the green vegetables.

15. Push your carbohydrate intake to later in the day and you will postpone that rush of insulin which stimulates your appetite and starts you on your eating course for the day.

16. Focus on food density. Eat foods that have a food density less than 4.

17. Don't eat the prison food! Make eating in restaurants work for you, not against you.

18. Make sure your carbohydrate intake matches your activity level: If you are sedentary, then limit your carbohydrates to less than 200 grams in a day. If you are physically active, you can venture up to 400. If you are trying to lose weight, shoot for only 100 grams.

19. Every meal counts.

20. Every time you sit down to eat, think PVC.

The Program

Now that you have been educated on the PVC Diet, you probably want to get started. The best place for you to go for more information is to our website: www.pvcdiet.com. We are building a repository of recipes and restaurant recommendations which are tailored to and driven by your specific carbohydrate needs. Weight loss is only one phase of your program. Weight maintenance is a lifelong process. We hope that our website will be a place for you to visit for ongoing assistance. Visit us at www.pvcdiet.com, on Facebook at PVC Diet and on Twitter @pvcdiet. Let's stay connected. Good luck!

About the Author

Lawrence R. Kosinski, MD, MBA has been a practicing Gastroenterologist for 30 years and is one of the founding partners of the Illinois Gastroenterology Group, the largest gastroenterology group in Illinois. He specializes in acid reflux (GERD), ulcers, diverticulosis, irritable bowel syndrome (IBS), Crohn's disease, ulcerative colitis and other digestive diseases. He believes nutrition is one of the most important issues to focus on to promote good health. Dr. Kosinski received his BS and MD from Loyola University, his MBA from Northwestern University Kellogg School of Business. He is a nationally recognized speaker and a Davies award recipient. He lives outside of Chicago with his wife Sherry and their puppy-mill rescued Chihuahuas—Valentino and Bluie.